PEDIATRIC EMERGENCIES

THOMAS F BEATTIE

MB FRCS (Ed.) FFAEM DCH

Consultant in Pediatric Accident and Emergency Care
Royal Hospital for Sick Children
Edinburgh, UK

G MICHAEL HENDRY

MB BS DMRD FRCR

Consultant Pediatric Radiologist
Royal Hospital for Sick Children
Edinburgh, UK

KEITH P DUGUID

FBIPP FRPS Hon FIMI

Director, Department of Medical Illustration
University of Aberdeen
Aberdeen, UK

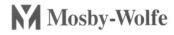 Mosby-Wolfe

London   Philadelphia   St. Louis   Sydney   Tokyo

Project Manager:	Leslie Sinoway
Development Editor:	Simon Pritchard
Designer:	Lara Last
Layout Artist:	Rob Curran
Cover Design:	Greg Smith
Cover Illustration:	Hamish Smith (aged 2 3/4)
Illustration:	Marion Tasker
Production:	Siobhan Egan
Index:	Anita Reid
Publisher:	Geoff Greenwood

ISBN 0 7234 1673 7

Copyright © 1997 Mosby-Wolfe. an imprint of Mosby International (a division of Times Mirror International Publishers Limited)

Published in 1997 by Mosby-Wolfe, an imprint of Mosby International (a division of Times Mirror International Publishers Limited)

Printed in Barcelona, Spain by Grafos S.A. Arte sobre papel, 1997

For full details of all Mosby International titles, please write to Mosby International, Lynton House, 7–12 Tavistock Square, London WC1H 9LB, UK.

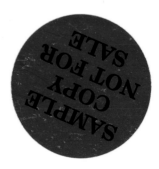

Contents

Preface

The identification and management of the sick and injured child requires special skills. While major illness or injury in children is relatively rare, the clinical situation can be fraught with anxiety and fear.

The management of the sick or injured child in the accident and emergency department requires a structured and orderly approach. The reactions of children to illness and trauma and the differing pathologies pertaining in pediatric practice make this a challenging specialty. As in other branches of medicine, excellent clinical skills are essential, but in pediatrics communication is of paramount importance. It is not enough to treat the child alone; parental (and even grandparental) anxiety has to be managed. *Pediatric Emergencies* arose from a need for an illustrated manual that junior doctors, medical students, and nursing staff could refer to in the accident and emergency department when dealing with the vast array of problems that present in the pediatric setting.

Individual practice may vary on both a geographical and a personal basis. We believe, however, that this book provides a safe and rational approach to the early management of the most common, and some rarer, conditions encountered by staff in the pediatric emergency department. Of course, it is not possible to illustrate every single condition, and factors involved in the choice of material include the availability of space, relevance to clinical practice, and personal preference. We hope that we have achieved a suitable balance.

This is a comprehensible illustrated text: descriptions of clinical procedures are enhanced through relevant photographs and diagrams, and key information is displayed in summary form in tables and charts. Throughout, topics are cross-referenced to ensure the reader is given as full a picture as possible. It is our hope that by presenting the book in this user-friendly fashion it will become a useful companion in the day-to-day practice of pediatric emergency care.

TFB
GMH
KPD
March 1997

Acknowledgements

We are deeply indebted to the many children and their parents who gave their permission for photographs to be taken. Without their consent this book would not have been possible.

We are grateful to the following for allowing us to reproduce material: Dr Angela Thomas, Consultant Haematologist, The Royal Hospital for Sick Children, Edinburgh (Fig. 3.39); The Department of Haematology, University of Aberdeen Medical School, Aberdeen (Fig. 3.38); and Dr Gaynor Cole, Consultant Paediatric Neurologist, Royal Aberdeen Children's Hospital, Aberdeen. Figures 5.17 and 5.19 are reproduced from: Spitz L *et al. Color Atlas of Pediatric Surgical Diagnosis*, Year Book Medical Publishers, Inc, Chicago, 1981.

Thanks are also extended to the staff of the radiography and medical illustration departments of The University of Aberdeen Medical School, Aberdeen, and The Royal Hospital for Sick Children, Edinburgh and the Aberdeen Royal Hospitals NHS Trust.

Finally, we wish to thank our families for their long-suffering tolerance of our participation in this project.

Chapter ONE

The Child and the Accident and Emergency Department

THE PEDIATRIC ACCIDENT AND EMERGENCY DEPARTMENT

Approximately 2.5 million children attend an Accident and Emergency Department (AED) in the UK annually. Most will have genuine cause to be in a hospital setting. Undoubtedly, many will have problems that could be treated in a community or general practice setting. There are many reasons why children attend AEDs; parental anxiety, availability of community services, access to primary health care and previous experience all play a part.

The role of the AED in the management of pediatric emergencies is to distinguish the child in need of emergency or urgent care from the large numbers of less serious presentations; to provide those children with an area where they can be best dealt with; and then to deal effectively with those children. This can be summarized as getting the right child to the right place to be treated by the right person in the right time frame.

The ability to treat any child at any given time will depend on the following factors:
- Number of children attending.
- Number of nursing staff.
- Number of medical staff.
- Availability of backup facilities.

This clearly requires a great deal of planning and preparation, a process facilitated by considering some important principles:
- Premises.
- Population served.

- Patterns of attendance.
- People.
- Preparation.
- Physical properties.
- Protocols.
- Priorities.
- Prevention.
- Practice review.

PREMISES

The environment within which pediatric accident and emergency medicine is practiced is important. Children are not young adults–they relate differently from adults to the outside world.

Common sense suggests that children are more amenable to treatment if they are calm and undistressed. A friendly, welcoming environment will help this (**Figure 1.1**). Every effort should be made to protect children from the sights and sounds of a typical adult accident and emergency setting. Ideally, children should be treated separately from the adult population by provision of separate waiting areas, treatment rooms and X-ray facilities (**Figures 1.2 and 1.3**). This, however, is not always possible. Even so, every effort should be made to protect the children as suggested above.

This can be facilitated by having bright, airy waiting rooms that have plenty of toys and games to keep the children occupied. The presence of a trained play leader in the accident and emergency setting has tremendous benefit.It is not just ill or injured children who benefit from play leaders or play therapy—parents can be relieved of some of the stress and worry occasioned by their ill or injured child. Parents may have to attend the AED accompanied by the

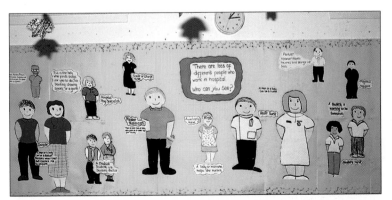

Figure 1.1
The environment where children are seen should be as welcoming as possible.

ill child's siblings whose needs will also have to be catered for. An active-play service within the AED waiting area can cater for the needs of these children leaving the parents or guardian to concentrate on the distressed or injured child (**Figure 1.4**).

The radiology suite must be close to all emergency services. At the very least standard X-ray units should be sited or planned close to the AED. Computerized tomography (CT), ultrasound or magnetic resonance imaging (MRI) may be necessary for evaluation of complex trauma and these facilities should be easily accessible from the AED. This will facilitate prompt care of the ill child in a facility close to the area where maximal resuscitation expertise is available.

Thus consideration should be given to having overhead X-ray equipment in the resuscitation room itself to facilitate plain radiography in ill or injured children without the need to transfer them to and from another part of the building. Portable X-ray units are a second-best choice.

Having intensive care and operating theatres adjacent to the emergency resuscitation room will also have a benefit in allowing rapid transfer of critically ill children to a place of definitive care. Proximity also allows staff more frequent meetings and informal collaboration, which can help to build teamwork and friendships.

To enable most children to benefit fully from the best facilities available, consideration should be given to centralizing pediatric emergency services at a base hospital. The base hospital should have a retrieval team to facilitate safe transfer of the ill or injured child to a central receiving area where resuscitation and treatment can be continued prior to transfer to imaging, theatre or intensive care. Having all the facilities required for the treatment of acute cases, i.e. theatres, intensive care, radiology and the emergency room, located adjacent to the receiving area will facilitate this.

The service will be complete if there is a facility to receive both land-based and helicopter transfers close to this receiving area.

Within the treatment setting, distraction therapy can again be employed. Familiar cartoon characters on the walls, toys and a friendly relaxed atmosphere can all help diagnosis and treatment (**Figure 1.5**).

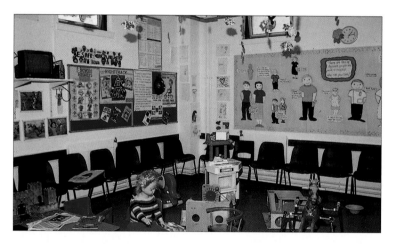

Figure 1.2
The waiting room should be child-friendly with toys and activities to amuse patients and siblings alike.

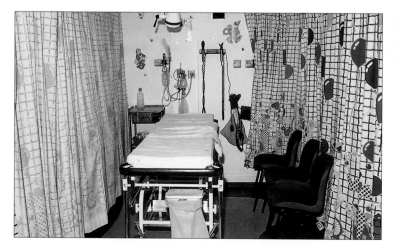

Figure 1.3
The treatment room well decorated with familiar figures can help to alleviate the fears of a distressed child.

Other facilities that can make the life of parents and children easier include nappy changing areas, areas where mothers can breastfeed in private and comfort and toilets dedicated to children (these should be of a height suitable for children to use on their own); these toilets should be exclusively for the use of children so they can be free from the attentions of undesirable adults.

It is a frequent misconception among lay-planners to think that pediatric facilities need to be smaller than adult facilities because children are smaller than adults. What is forgotten is that the staff working in both areas are the same shape and size (**Figure 1.6**)! In addition, children are often accompanied by an extended family, making, if anything, the needs of children, in terms of space, greater.

POPULATION SERVED

All of us know that children grow and develop from birth to adulthood. One of the debates of modern times is when to stop treating children in pediatric facilities. Is it at puberty? Is it at the age of 16 or 18? Local policies and practice will determine the needs of the individual and place them in the appropriate facility accordingly.

It is important for these issues to be addressed and decisions made. The needs of the adolescent population are different to those of the infant and toddler group. New pathologies start to emerge which necessitate a different way of thinking. Pregnancy has to be considered in the adolescent presenting with abdominal pain; poisoning in the adolescent is seldom accidental; fractures in the adolescent may not remodel to the same degree as in the younger child.

If teenagers and adolescents are to be seen and treated in a 'pediatric' facility then their emotional and psychological needs must be met in an appropriate way.

In Scotland, it is generally accepted that the appropriate time to transfer children to an adult facility is around the time of puberty. This does not stop immature children attending a pediatric facility but will encourage mature and peri- and postpubertal children to be dealt with in facilities more used to dealing with adults.

The catchment area of the department will have an impact on the needs of the population. Poor, socio-economically deprived areas place a higher demand on all services than do more affluent areas. It is easier to discharge equivocal cases if home circumstances are good.

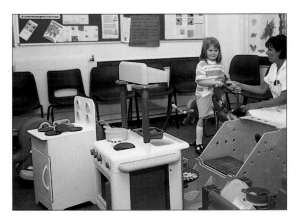

Figure 1.4
A child playing in the waiting room supervised by a member of staff, so allowing the parents to comfort her injured sibling.

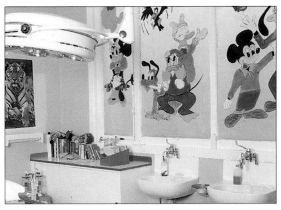

Figure 1.5
Familiar characters can help make the child more relaxed and make the atmosphere friendlier.

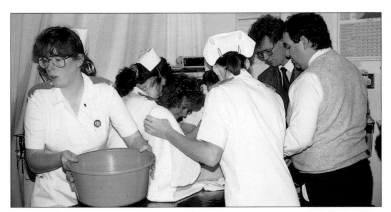

Figure 1.6
A large number of people are often needed to help in pediatric resuscitation. Space is important.

Rural and urban areas also have different requirements. Transport to and from hospital can be difficult for each group, but for different reasons. All of these factors will have to be considered in planning the needs for a given community.

PATTERNS OF ATTENDANCE

The spectrum of disease and injury is vast, but certain attendance patterns emerge when analyzed over time. There are both seasonal and temporal variations in this pattern. In the UK, pediatric trauma reaches its peak in the summer months but respiratory disease is more prevalent in the winter months. Other conditions show no such seasonal trends but present at any time of the year. Some accidents are equally prevalent throughout the year, e.g. burns and poisoning.

Daily variations also occur. The morning can often be relatively quiet, attendances reaching a plateau sometime after lunch. A steady state then exists until about 5 p.m. when another mini peak occurs with attendances eventually falling-off towards midnight (**Figure 1.7**).

A knowledge of these typical patterns is essential to enable planning of the service. The knock-on effect from a busy medical service in the winter months will put pressure on the medical wards. Similarly, accidents and other

trauma will put pressure on the surgical services during the summer months. These factors should be taken into consideration when planning work loads on both the medical and surgical sides. Failure to address these needs will lead to bed-blocking, uneven staffing and frustration all round.

PEOPLE

Staffing in pediatric emergency care is crucial. Dealing with pediatric emergencies can be one of the most worrying and frightening experiences but, when successful, one of the most rewarding. Staff working with children must enjoy the challenge. They must be comfortable with children and be aware of the different needs of the growing child; this 'comfort' relates to both clinical and psychological matters. The best facilities in the world will be wasted otherwise.

All senior staff within the emergency department should have training in the skills required to deal effectively with children. This will help to create an ambience suitable for the training of junior staff, who will hopefully become imbued with the correct ethos, thus creating a self-perpetuating quality of care.

It should also be borne in mind that one is not only treating children but also the guardians and relatives of

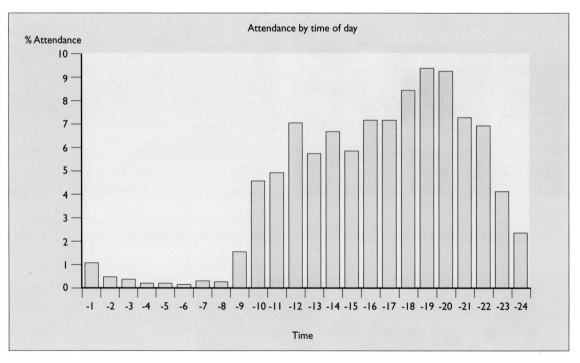

Figure 1.7
Typical pattern of attendance at an AED over a 24-hour period.

children presenting to the department. Very often the parents need as much time and consideration as the child and staff within the AED should recognize and provide this.

PREPARATION

In all emergency situations forewarned is forearmed. Unfortunately, in emergency pediatric practice this cannot always be so.

Pediatric practice is different to adult practice where prehospital services are more frequently involved. In the situation where ambulances are needed there is usually warning given. This allows time to assemble a team, allocate tasks and mentally prepare for the work in hand. As some indication of the cause of the problem will have been communicated earlier, protocols can be discussed with junior staff to help them perform their tasks—this is not possible with a moribund infant carried in its mother's arms.

Despite this, the AED should be able to respond appropriately whether it be to a single child or to a major disaster involving many children.

Preparation will involve equipment, both for resuscitation and otherwise; staffing and training issues; protocols and guidelines; and lines of communication. Where relevant these will be addressed in the chapters which follow.

The equipment in the acute areas, such as the resuscitation room and critical-care areas, needs to be adaptable for use in the treatment of children of all ages. This is not a problem in combined adult and pediatric units. In pediatric units, however, it is not uncommon to be asked to deal with adults, often either relatives or staff, who may be in need of urgent care and this possibility should be catered for.

Cervical collars of suitable size are hard to find for small children. One answer is to improvise as shown below (**Figures** 1.8–1.9).

Mobility is compromised in children with an injured lower limb. Wheelchairs appropriate to the age of the child can be helpful (**Figure** 1.10). Older children can manage crutches with practice but younger children, especially those between 3 and 5 years of age, find crutches difficult to use. They are often too heavy for parents to carry around with comfort, especially if a long leg cast is needed and they are too young and uncoordinated to use crutches. These factors must be addressed prior to a child being discharged.

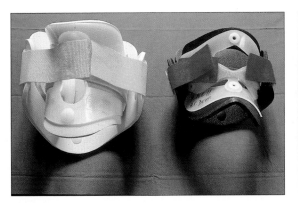

Figure 1.8
Typical commercial hard collars available for children. The smaller size does not fit very small children. Although the chance of cervical-spine injury is low, these collars are inadequate for small children.

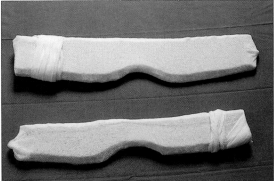

Figure 1.9
It may be necessary to create hard collars as shown here. These, however, do not stop full movement and an additional method of support is needed if cervical-spine injury is suspected.

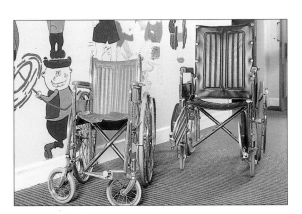

Figure 1.10
Wheelchairs of different sizes. The larger type will be needed for adolescents.

PHYSICAL PROPERTIES

The priorities of pediatric emergency care revolve around the 'ABC of resuscitation'. The principles of resuscitation are the same for children as for adults but the actual practice in children is complicated because resuscitation procedures change with age.

ANATOMICAL DIFFERENCES

Babies and toddlers have a relatively large head compared to the older child. This gives the child a slightly top heavy centre of gravity making head injury one of the more common injuries in childhood.

Associated with the large head is a relatively large occiput. This can make airway-opening maneuvers difficult and can affect intubation techniques.

Other factors that influence pediatric airway care include:

- Large tongue.
- Floppy epiglottis.
- Narrow-based epiglottis.
- Relatively high larynx.
- Narrow point at the cricoid cartilage.

These all combine to make intubation in babies and young children a different process to that used in the older child or adult. For those used to these factors, airway care is easy; for occasional practitioners the differences can prove insurmountable.

Further points in the head region that make therapy difficult include the presence of sutures and fontanelles; these can make interpretation of skull fractures difficult for the inexperienced—indeed, even for the experienced there is sometimes debate as to whether a given line on a skull X-ray is a suture, fracture or vascular marking (**Figure 1.11**)! The presence of sutures and fontanelles means that expanding cranial lesions do not necessarily have the same pressure

effects in children as they have in older people. A high index of suspicion is therefore needed to help determine the presence or absence of intracranial lesions in young children.

Within the chest the most important anatomic difference is the position of the heart. The heart in infants is situated much higher in the chest than in older children and adults. This influences the hand position for cardiac massage and other invasive procedures involving the heart (*see* Chapter 3, hand position).

The rib cage is not entirely protective of the liver and spleen in the smaller infant. In trauma situations therefore these organs are disproportionately more frequently damaged than in the older child—this is particularly true in non-accidental injury.

In infants and small children various anatomical remnants may give rise to pathology not usually typical of the older child and adult. For example a patent urachus may give rise to discharging lesions around the umbilicus in young children.

The biggest difference in the child skeleton is in the structure of the bones. Bones in children are a mixture of cartilage and bone. The cartilage will develop in time into fully mature bone. Until such time as this occurs injury to the cartilage, particularly around the epiphyseal regions, may be invisible on a plain X-ray. Formal classification of epiphyseal injuries can be found in the orthopedic section.

Children's bones are different to those of adults as they are more pliable and have a thicker periosteum. The flexibility of children's bones means that children are prone to a condition called plastic deformation where the bone may actually bend without fracturing (**Figure 1.12** and *see* Orthopedic section).

The thicker periosteum means that bones heal more quickly when fractured and this reduces the time for therapeutic intervention such as manipulation. The bonus is that bones in childhood are often very resilient.

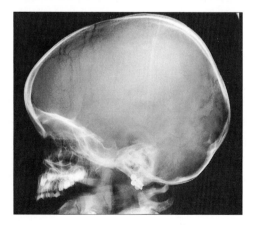

Figure 1.11
Lateral skull Xray demonstrating prominent vascular markings in the frontal region of the vault. These are not to be confused with fracture lines. Vascular markings are usually curvilinear, less radiolucent than fractures and have slightly sclerotic margins.

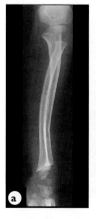 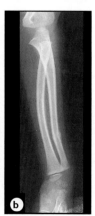

Figure 1.12 b
A film 10 days later shows healing of the ulnar fracture and periosteal reaction along the radial shaft indicating a healing cortical injury.

Figure 1.12 a
Oblique views of the forearm. in a child suffering a fall on the out-stretched hand. There is a fracture of the distal ulnar diaphysis and associated plastic bowing of the radius.

Remodeling may occur despite inappropriate anatomic alignment (*see* **Figure 1.12** on previous page). Fractures in the midshaft of the bone are unlikely to remodel as effectively as those located proximally and distally.

The nature of the blood supply to the growth plate in children makes it more prone to acute hematogenous osteomyelitis than in the older population (Chapter 5).

PHYSIOLOGICAL DIFFERENCES

Beginning with the head, babies are obligate nose breathers. This persists up to almost 1 year of age. Respiratory rates change with age (**Figure 1.13a**). Respiratory distress in children is manifested by an increasing respiratory rate, increasing use of accessory and intercostal muscles, sternal and intercostal recession and a decreasing level of consciousness (*see* Chapter 2).

The presence of cyanosis is an unreliable sign and greater emphasis should be placed on other clinical signs.

The pliability of the pediatric rib cage enables tremendous recession to take place with a sometimes dramatic appearance. In the chest, the ribs are springier making fracture much more difficult.

Similarly, the blood pressure and pulse rate change with age; there is a wide variation within each of these (**Figures 1.12 and 1.13**).

In hypovolemic situations children have a tremendous ability to compensate by peripheral vasoconstriction. This diverts the blood flow from the peripheral and non-vital areas to vital areas. Up to 50% of the blood volume in a child can be lost before blood pressure will actually fall. This means that blood pressure is an extremely unreliable indicator of the clinical status of a child (Chapter 2).

NEUROLOGICAL DEVELOPMENT

Developmental delay in a child is an important factor in many situations. Often it will be picked up as part of a routine developmental assessment. More often it has been present from birth as a result of obstetric problems. In particular, children should have lost neonatal reflexes and gained new skills as they get older (**Figure 1.14**).

A child who has previously developed normally, but who regresses should be taken seriously. There may well be an underlying organic cause such as a neurological problem. However, the need may be emotional and may indeed be a harbinger of either physical or sexual abuse.

Whatever the cause, an assessment of the child's developmental stages should always be made when in the accident and emergency setting (**Figure 1.15**). This will be informal in most cases, but where there is cause for concern a more formal examination should be carried out.

Assessment of consciousness can be difficult in small children. The Glasgow Coma Scale is probably only suitable for children aged 5 years and older (*see* Trauma chapter) . Many scales exist, all of which give some indication of the level of consciousness and help with continued assessment. It is recommended that a unit uses one system consistently.

Age	Range	Mean
Birth–3 Months	30–40	35
3 Months–1 Year	20–35	30
1–5 Years	20–30	25
5–10 Years	15–25	20
>10 Years	12–15	14

Figure 1.13 a Respiratory rates by age

Reflex	Age lost
Moro	3 Months
Palmar grasp	4 Months
Rooting	8 Months

Figure 1.14 Typical age at which early reflexes are lost.

Age	Mean blood pressure mmHg
Birth	60/40
1 Year	95/65
5 Years	100/65
Puberty	120/75

Figure 1.13 b Mean blood pressure values for different age groups

Age	Mean heart rate (beats/min)
Birth	125
1 Year	125
5 Years	100
Puberty	75

Figure 1.13 c Mean heart rates for different age groups.

Age	Verbal skill developed	Motor skill developed
3 Months	Has startle response	Wriggles
6 Months	Babbles	Rolls over
8 Months	Responds to name	Crawls
12 Months	Understands words	Walks Holding on
18 Months	Says "mama" and "dada"	Climbs stairs
36 Months	Uses short sentences	Runs, uses tricycle

Figure 1.15 Some typical milestones in child development grouped by age.

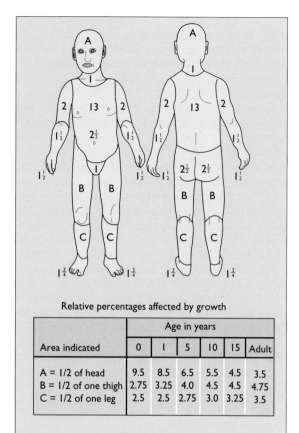

Relative percentages affected by growth

Area indicated	Age in years					
	0	1	5	10	15	Adult
A = 1/2 of head	9.5	8.5	6.5	5.5	4.5	3.5
B = 1/2 of one thigh	2.75	3.25	4.0	4.5	4.5	4.75
C = 1/2 of one leg	2.5	2.5	2.75	3.0	3.25	3.5

Figure 1.16
Burns chart showing the difference in surface areas of different parts of the body in different age groups.

SURFACE AREA DIFFERENCES

Children, proportional to their height, have a larger surface area than adults. Clinically this is important because young children will lose heat more rapidly than older individuals. This is relevant in the resuscitation room where care must be taken to avoid prolonged exposure during examinations and procedures.

Patients with burns are assessed according to surface area. A typical burns assessment chart is shown opposite. This indicates the relative surface areas according to age (**Figure 1.16**).

PROPORTIONAL DIFFERENCES

The varying dimensions of children at various stages of life have already been discussed. It would be very useful if every child presenting as an emergency was able to tell us their exact height and weight; unfortunately, this is not the case. In order to adequately treat children it is necessary to have a ready approximate method for calculation available—this can be done using either a a tape or chart. Either should be available on every resuscitation cart or within the resuscitation area and should be used until more accurate information is available (**Figures 1.17and 1.18**).

In the absence of these aids, an approximate weight can be calculated as follows:

$$\text{Weight in kg} = (\text{age} \times 2) + 8$$

This is valid up to about 8–10 years of age.

PROTOCOLS

The management of pediatric emergencies should follow set practices determined prior to the child arriving. These will give a framework for junior and inexperienced staff to practice safe, immediate care. Within this framework there should be a recommendation that senior staff should be

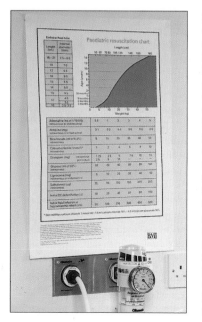

Figure 1.17
Chart showing the relationship between bodyweight and age based upon the 50th centile weight. In addition, information is presented to enable rapid approximate calculation of drug and fluid volumes together with appropriate endotracheal tube size and length. It should be prominently displayed on a wall in the resuscitation room.

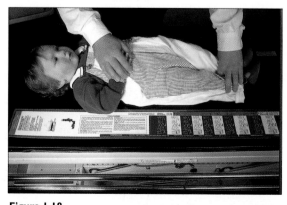

Figure 1.18
Use of a linear tape measure to calculate the same information as shown in Figure 1.17.

called to help and advise with difficult cases. As a general rule these protocols should be adhered to in the first instance and only varied by senior advice. In addition, basic advice should be available to help with the management of difficult areas such as suspected child abuse and sudden infant death syndrome.

PRIORITIES

As mentioned at the beginning of the chapter, the numbers of children attending AEDs is large, and growing. Unfortunately, it is not possible to see each of these children as soon as they arrive. A system of prioritization (**Triage**) is therefore necessary.

TRIAGE

Triage involves the identification of the urgency with which children require treatment, placing them in the appropriate category, and then allocating the resources available to deal with the child in the appropriate time frame. It is an inexact science which deals with many variables. Correct triage will depend on the experience of the triage staff and adherence to objective directions. Subconscious pressures to under-triage (i.e. allocate to a less urgent category) occur when the department is busy and vice versa when the department is quiet.

TRIAGE CATEGORIES
1 Resuscitation
The resuscitation category includes children who are in cardiopulmonary failure or cardiac arrest. These children need to be seen, assessed and treated *on arrival* by the most experienced staff available.

2 Emergency
Children falling into the emergency category will be in shock or severe respiratory distress. Delay in their treatment should be minimal and should really only be preceded by those children in category 1.

3 Urgent
Urgent cases should be seen next after categories 1 and 2. Children who fall into this category include those in mild–moderate respiratory distress, dehydration and pain.

4 Non-urgent
The final category is cases who are non-urgent. These children will be seen only after all other categories have been dealt with. These children can wait for treatment and many could in fact be treated in the community but have presented to the AED.

Triage is a dynamic process. Once placed in a given triage category the child should be regularly re-assessed to determine if he or she needs to be moved up or down a category.

Parents are in the emergency room because they are concerned for their child. This concern will often cause them to be abusive if they see other, though probably more urgent cases, being treated first. Communication and explanation of the triage system are therefore needed.

PREVENTION
Many childhood diseases and injuries are preventable. The AED is ideally placed to play a part in preventive medicine. No other service has such a large captive population from whom to assess the prevention needs of the community. Information regarding immunization rates and uptake can be monitored; accident risk can be evaluated, e.g. use of cycle helmets; problem areas can be identified from computerized records of accident black-spots. Awareness of this facility is important if strides to a safer environment for children are to be made (**Figure 1.19**).

PRACTICE REVIEW (AUDIT)

Practice review is an important part of clinical practice. Within pediatric accident and emergency care, which is a very young specialty, many issues need to be addressed. The continued questioning of current practice, by audit and research, is vital to the development of the specialty; without it we cannot hope to achieve improvements in the currently high rates of mortality and morbidity from cardiac arrest in childhood.

By constantly evaluating miss-fracture rates, underdiagnosis, overtreatment and failures of the system the care of each individual child will improve.

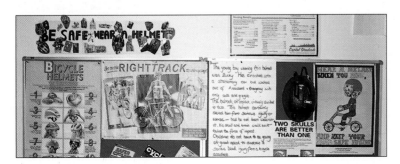

Figure 1.19
An 'accident prevention' corner within an AED setting. This poster demonstrates the benefits of using cycle helmets.

INITIAL ASSESSMENT AND MANAGEMENT OF THE CHILD

RECOGNITION OF THE SICK CHILD

One of the major skills necessary for the safe practice of emergency pediatric care is the ability to recognize the child whose condition is potentially life-threatening. The individual list of diseases that can cause life-threatening illness is vast. but, with few exceptions, these have a common pathway (**Figure 1.20**).

RESPIRATORY FAILURE

Respiratory failure is the end-point of a prolonged disease process. Typically, it is preceded by a period of either decreased or increased respiratory effort. Decreased respiratory effort is usually associated with conditions out-with the lungs and airway. Increased respiratory effort is usually associated with airway and lung disease. In both cases the net result is an inability to maintain oxygenation leading to gradual and progressive hypoxia and concomitant retention of carbon dioxide.

Increased work of breathing

This is probably the most common of respiratory difficulties among children. Typically, there is narrowing of the airways either due to infection, inflammation or foreign body impaction; occasionally all three coexist. The child finds it increasingly hard to maintain normal oxygen levels and its body works overtime to try and achieve this. Increased muscular effort is required, resulting in the use of intercostal and accessory muscles and a generalized increase in respiratory rate (**Figure 1.21**). Gradual loss of consciousness occurs as hypoxia ensues (**Figure 1.22**).

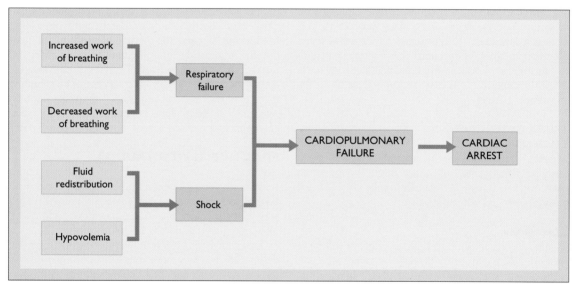

Figure 1.20 Common final pathway for hypoxia and hypovolaemia.

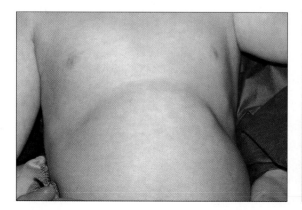

Figure 1.21
Child demonstrating increased work of breathing with marked intercostal recession.

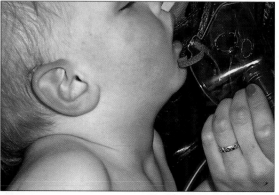

Figure 1.22
A child with severe respiratory distress. The child is not fully awake and has extended his neck to the sniffing position and is using his accessory muscles.

The ability to maintain increased respiratory effort is dependent on the amount of energy available. An inability to take in fluids and energy is usually associated with increased work of breathing. The child is therefore dependent on its glycogen stores which are very much lower in an infant than in an older child. Gradually, as the glycogen stores are used up and muscle fatigue sets in, the ability to maintain the effort required diminishes until the child goes into respiratory failure.

In addition, as the child becomes exhausted, hypoxia increases, which in turn aggravates the ability of the muscles to work.

It is imperative therefore to recognize a child in whom the work of breathing is increasing and to intervene aggressively (**Figure 1.23**).

Decreased respiration

As mentioned above, decreased respiration is usually associated with factors outwith the lungs and airway. Restrictive forces may be placed on the lung tissue by pneumothorax, hemothorax or gastric dilatation. Central causes, e.g. head injury, poisoning and other neurological disorders, cause hypoventilation. In all these situations the airway must be opened and usually some form of assisted ventilation is required. Treatable causes such as gastric dilatation must also be addressed. It is important to

recognize the child who is making an inadequate respiratory effort and to take therapeutic measures.

Respiratory depression may have an insidious onset. Underlying disease may lead to coma which in turn leads to respiratory depression (**Figure 1.24**). The subsequent hypoxia will often aggravate the respiratory depression, thus developing into a vicious cycle. Such cases may be detected not by increasing respiratory effort but by signs of hypoxia. Prime among these is altered mentation, confusion and agitation. The respiratory rate will often be slow with the depth of breathing shallow.

As a rule of thumb, where it is difficult to determine cause and effect, oxygen saturation should be measured and, oxygen applied by a face mask initially and by bag/valve/mask if necessary. A response by either rising oxygen saturation, improved mentation or both, is an indication for continued therapy.

HYPOVOLEMIA

Hypovolemia is associated with many conditions. (**Figure 1.25**). Probably the most common cause world-wide are gastro enteritis and trauma. No matter what the cause of the hypovolemia, the child will rapidly begin to develop circulatory compromise if the underlying cause is not rapidly recognized and treated. As hypovolemia worsens, the body attempts to compensate for the circulatory deficit by

---

Increasing respiratory effort is characterized by:
• Open mouth
• Nasal flaring
• Neck extension
• Use of accessory muscles
• Intercostal recession
• Sternal recession
• Altered level of consciousness

Figure 1.23

Obstructive	Restrictive	Neuromuscular	External/central
Foreign body	Pneumothorax	Spinal injury	Head injury
Bronchiolitis	Hemothorax	Polio	Poisoning
Asthma	Gastric	Guillain-Barré	Coma
Epiglottitis	dilatation	Spinal cord	
Croup	Rib injury (pain)	tumors	
Tracheitis			

Figure 1.24 Classification of underlying diseases responsible for respiratory distress and failure.

Fluid loss	Redistribution
Diarrhea	Sepsis
Vomiting	Cardiac failure
Hemorrhage	Neurogenic shock
Diabetic	Anaphylaxis
ketoacidosis	

Figure 1.25 Conditions which can lead to Hypovolemia.

constricting the peripheral circulation in an effort to maintain perfusion to the vital organs in the chest and brain. There are signs associated with this peripheral shutdown. (**Figures 1.26 and 1.27a–c**).

The history is vital to determine the underlying cause of the problem. This should only be taken in detail after the child is safe and resuscitation is under way. Additional physical signs of note should be sought, e.g. a petechial rash may be found in meningococcemia (this is not always florid) (*see* The Ill Child, Chapter 4.)

It is important therefore to recognize these early signs and to take corrective action. Failure to do so will lead to a child going into decompensated shock which will rapidly progress to cardiopulmonary failure and possibly cardiac arrest (**Figure 1.20**).

Having recognized that the child is ill it is now appropriate to take measures to treat the child. A structured approach to care is necessary. Traditionally, one uses the 'ABCD' of resuscitation, which prioritizes care in a logical sequence (**Figure 1.28**); in detail this is used as follows.

1. AIRWAY

ASSESSMENT OF THE PEDIATRIC AIRWAY
The pediatric airway can be described as **normal, maintainable** or **unmaintainable**. The airway should be described as being normal only if the child is fully alert and there is adequate air flow.

A maintainable airway is one which can be kept clear by simple techniques such as suction, positioning (e.g. recovery position) or by chin lift/head tilt measures.

An unmaintainable airway is one which requires intubation or the creation of a surgical airway.

MAINTENANCE OF THE PEDIATRIC AIRWAY
The single most important airway maneuver is the **chin lift/head tilt** (**Figure 1.29**). Care must be taken not to compress soft tissues in the submental area. Fingers must be placed on the mandible to avoid compressing the soft tissues in the floor of the mouth, consequently aggravating

---

Altered level of consciousness
Absent peripheral pulses
Wide toe–core temperature difference
Increasing capillary return (>2 secs)
Decreasing urine output

Figure 1.26 Clinical signs of shock

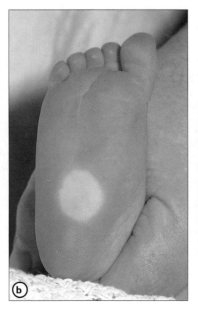
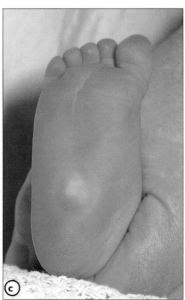

Figure 1.27
(a) Capillary-refill test. The leg is raised slightly and the examiner's finger pressed for a few seconds on the sole of the foot.

(b) A clear imprint of the finger remains. In normal circumstances the imprint should disappear in under 2 seconds.
(c) There is still an imprint visible after 8 seconds, indicating severe circulatory compromise.

airway obstruction. Gentle suction can help remove liquid and particularly matter from the oropharynx. A rigid Yankauer suction catheter is best.(**Figure** 1.30).

A Guedel airway may be needed to augment the airway opening. The correct size has a length corresponding to the distance between the lips and the angle of the mandible. (**Figure** 1.31; *see also* Chapter 2).

Definitive care of the airway is usually secured by intubation, a skill that needs training and practice. A laryngoscope in the wrong hands has been described as an 'oxygen deprivation device'.

In infants, the trachea should be intubated using uncuffed endotracheal tubes. Older children, usually between 8–9 years of age, and certainly those approaching puberty, will require cuffed tubes, so a selection should always be available. The narrow point at the cricoid in young children enables the uncuffed tracheal tube to fit snugly into the trachea without any additional space-filling device, i.e. a balloon. In older children, the narrowest point in the airway is the glottis, necessitating a tube that can pass through the glottic folds and then be expanded in the cavern below to ensure a snug fit and a sealed airway.

A -	Airway
B -	Breathing
C -	Circulation
D -	Disability

Figure 1.28 Priorities of care in ill or injured children

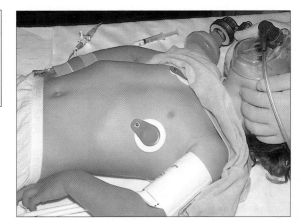

Figure 1.29
Chin lift/head tilt is an important method of securing the pediatric airway. Care must be taken not to put the large fingers of the resuscitator's hand into the relatively small area and soft tissues behind the mandible.

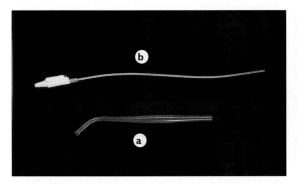

Figure 1.30
Two types of suction catheters are available: (a) a rigid Yankauer sucker and (b) a more flexible type. Yankauer suckers are more useful for removing vomit and other secretions from the pharynx.

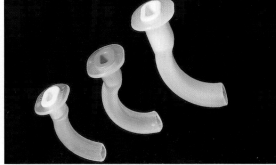

Figure 1.31
Guedel airways come in various sizes. It is important to choose a size appropriate for the child.

There are a variety of methods to identify the correct diameter of tube to be used (**Figure 1.32**); none are completely accurate, so a range of sizes must be available (**Figure 1.33**).

ORAL INTUBATION

Before starting, all equipment must be checked (**Figure 1.34**). For infants and younger children a straight-bladed laryngoscope is preferable–older children may require a curved blade.

Technique

The head should be placed in the sniffing position and bag/valve/mask ventilation should be continued until all the equipment is ready. The laryngoscope should be held in the left hand and brought into the pharynx, slowly while bringing the tongue out of the way. If using a straight-bladed laryngoscope, the epiglottis should be visualized and then lifted straight up. It is sometimes helpful to think about bringing the hand towards the opposite corner of the room. If a curved blade is used it should be slipped into the vallecula and lifted in the same direction as a straight-bladed laryngoscope (**Figure 1.35**).

The vocal cords should then come into view.

Occasionally, fluid and mucus are present. These should be gently sucked away under direct vision with a Yankauer sucker. Once the vocal cords are clearly in view, the endotracheal tube should be taken in the right hand and passed through the cords. It is important not to push the tube down too far. Most endotracheal tubes have a mark indicating when they have gone through the vocal cords.

Once the tube is in the trachea it should be attached to a bag/valve/mask device. This should be gently compressed and the operator should listen for air entry to both axillae with a stethoscope. Once there is bilateral air entry, the operator should firmly tape the tube into position in order to avoid it slipping down the trachea or falling into the esophagus. The complications of intubation are illustrated in **Figure 1.36** opposite.

NASAL INTUBATION

Almost exactly the same procedure is used for nasal intubation, the only difference being that the tube is passed down through the nose, from which position attempts are made to pass the tube through the cords. It is often necessary to use Magill's forceps to facilitate passage of the tube through the vocal cords.

Methods for determining the correct endotracheal tube
1. Endotracheal tube = (age +16)/4 = internal diameter
2. Width of child's little fingernail
3. A.P. Diameter of child's little finger
4. Width of child's little finger

Figure 1.32

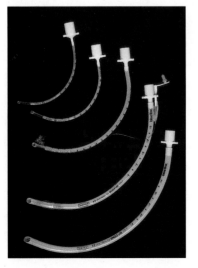

Figure 1.33
Different sized endotracheal tubes demonstrating cuffed and uncuffed varieties.

Equipment needed for intubation
1. Laryngoscope
2. Correctly sized ET tube
3. ET tube cut to correct length*
4. Suction device, tubing and suckers
5. Appropriately sized introducer
6. Bag-valve-mask device and connectors
7. Stethoscope
8. An assistant who is able to apply cricoid pressure and assist with ventilation

Figure 1.34
*Some practitioners prefer to leave tubes uncut.

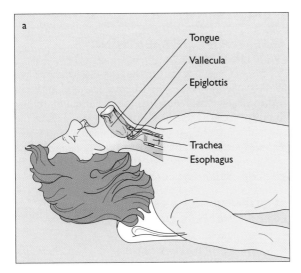

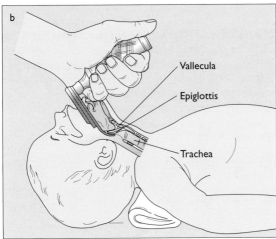

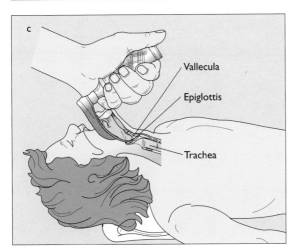

Figure 1.35

Intubation

(a) Normal anatomy

(b) Method of intubation using a straight-bladed laryngoscope in an infant

(c) Method of intubation using a curved-laryngoscope blade in an older child.

CREATION OF A SURGICAL (ARTIFICIAL) AIRWAY

In some circumstances, including upper airway obstruction, it is impossible or even dangerous to contemplate oral intubation. In these situations it is necessary to create a surgical airway rapidly and simply.

The simplest way to do this is by needle cricothyroidotomy (**Figures 1.37–1.41**). The technique for cricothyroid puncture is as follows:

- Continue attempts to ventilate using bag/valve/mask.
- Have all equipment ready.
- Rapidly clean the front of the child's neck with disinfectant.
- Position the child with a small towel under the shoulders and gently extend the neck.
- Attach a cannula and needle to a syringe.
- Ensure the rubber bung on the syringe is not stuck.
- Palpate the cricothyroid membrane below the thyroid cartilage in the midline.
- Gently insert the needle and cannula into the membrane while drawing back on the syringe.
- A sudden give will be felt and air will be aspirated into the syringe when the trachea is entered.
- Advance the cannula over the needle further into the trachea (air movement will be seen and heard only if respiratory effort is present).
- Attach the connector and bag/valve/mask to cannula.
- Attempt to ventilate **with gentle pressure**.

This technique will allow oxygen to be delivered but will not achieve effective alveolar ventilation; carbon dioxide levels will rise over a period of time. This method will buy time until intubation can be achieved. However, the technique is not without its problems and complications (*see* **Figure 1.41** overleaf).

Potential complications of intubation

1. Failure to intubate within 45 seconds will lead to hypoxia
2. Intubation of the right (or left) main bronchus
3. Intubation of the esophagus
4. Local trauma if the intubation attempt is not very gentle

Figure 1.36

Equipment for emergency cricothyroid puncture

1. Cannula over hollow needle
2. Syringe
3. Connectors
4. Appropriate ventilation equipment

Figure 1.37

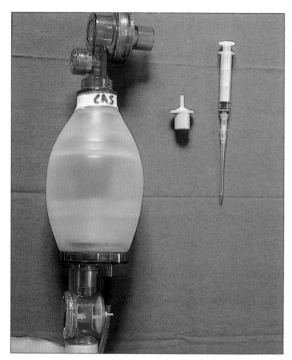

Figure 1.38
Basic equipment for cricothyroid puncture. There is debate over the method of ventilation. Some operators recommend a bag-valve-mask (as pictured here); others favor a jet insufflation device.

2. BREATHING

ASSESSMENT OF BREATHING (VENTILATION)

Adequacy of breathing can only be assessed after the airway has been opened. There should be evidence of clear, unobstructed air entry with no gurgling or other sounds during air entry or exit. The chest should be examined for the rate and depth of chest wall excursion and also the symmetry of movement. Both sides of the chest should be auscultated to ensure that air entry is full throughout both lung fields and that no pneumothorax is present.

SEQUENCE FOR ASSESSING EFFECTIVENESS OF VENTILATION

- Ensure that the airway is open.
- Look, listen and feel for air entry.
- Check for symmetry of movement.
- Listen for full air entry.

MAINTENANCE OF VENTILATION

As already mentioned, infants are obligate nose breathers. In childhood, normal respiratory rates vary with age making single assessment of respiratory rate practically meaningless. Of more importance is the rate over time. In the first instance, artificial ventilation should aim to mimic normal patterns for children.

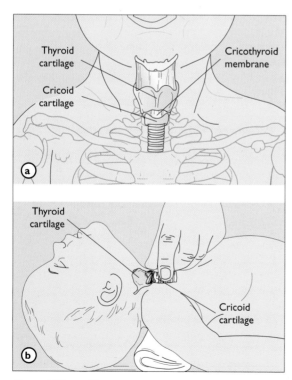

Figure 1.39 a and b
(a) Anatomical structures important for cricothyroidotomy.
(b) Lateral view of neck anatomy before procedure. Index finger and thumb identify cricoid cartilage.

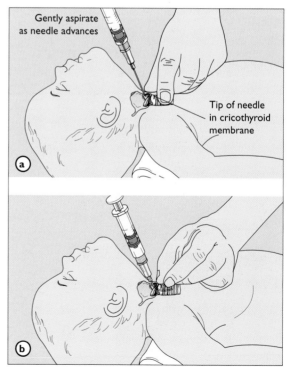

Figure 1.40 a and b
(a) Having identified cricothyroid membrane the cannula is gently introduced.
(b) When the airway is entered air will be drawn into the syringe. The cannula can be pushed into the trachea.

Effective artificial ventilation may be achieved using a **bag/valve/mask** device. A range of masks are available: clear, black, triangular, round etc. there are arguments for and against each. Round masks are easier to use in infants and younger children, particularly for occasional users. Clear masks offer, theoretically, a better view of vomitus.

At least two sizes of self-inflating bags should be available. The smaller one illustrated in **Figure 1.42** is adequate for all small children including neonates. The larger bag is for use in older children and adults.

The pediatric bag/valve/mask device, shown in **Figure 1.42**, differs in several ways to the type used in older children and adults. A 'pop-off' valve is inserted close to the one-way valve. The purpose of the valve is to avoid over-inflating the lungs in a small child a process which can result in barotrauma. Typically, the valve will 'blow' at pressures of 30–40 cm water thereby protecting the lungs. In situations where airway resistance may be high, the valve may blow at pressures lower than the airway pressure so necessitating manual compression of the valve before ventilation will be effective.

Both sizes of bag will deliver 100% oxygen only if:
- The seal around the mask is good.
- The bag is connected to an oxygen supply.
- A reservoir bag is fitted.

Complications of creating a surgical airway

1. Penetration of the esophagus
2. Surgical emphysema
3. Hemorrhage
4. Failure to establish oral airway

Figure 1.41

Otherwise lower concentrations of oxygen will be delivered, often insufficient to meet the demands of a shocked, collapsed or compromised child.

More experienced operators (e.g. anesthetists) may prefer an Ayre's T-piece circuit which gives a better feel of the compliance and ventilation. Use of this equipment requires practice and it is often difficult for the occasional operator to master (**Figure 1.43**). It is recommended that both the bag/valve/mask and T-piece circuits be made available to cater for individual preference.

The tidal volume is usually 7–10 ml/Kg. This is usually difficult to measure accurately in emergency situations. On each breath, the chest wall should be seen to rise and fall. Ventilation pressure should be sufficient for the chest wall to rise and no more.

TENSION PNEUMOTHORAX

Tension pneumothorax is a critical emergency that is potentially life-threatening. As it gets bigger it decreases the available area of the lung for gas exchange and oxygenation. Similarly, it interferes with venous return and cardiac output.

The clinical signs of a tension pneumothorax include:
- Respiratory distress and insufficiency.
- Distended neck veins.
- Decreased breath sounds on the affected side.
- Increased resonance on the affected side.

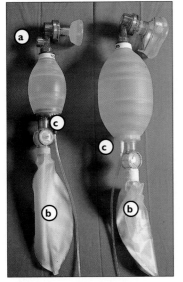

Figure 1.42
Bag/valve/mask devices suitable for use in children. The smaller bag on the left is appropriate for infants and younger children. It has a pop-off valve (a) which the large bag lacks. Both have a facility to supply 100% oxygen by way of reservoir bags (b). The oxygen is delivered at point (c). In order to deliver 100% oxygen the flow rate must be compatible with the manufacturer's recommendations.

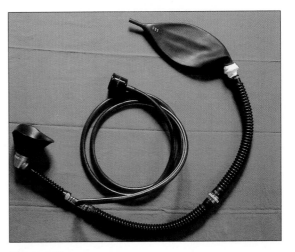

Figure 1.43
A typical anesthetic circuit often preferred by anesthetists.

There is no place for diagnosis by X-ray. It is a clinical diagnosis and must be treated as a matter of urgency.

TREATMENT
The child should be placed on supplemental high-flow oxygen. The tension pneumothorax should be immediately decompressed by inserting a large bore needle into the second intercostal space in the midclavicular line (**Figure 1.44**). A large hiss of air indicates that the diagnosis is correct and the patient's condition should improve as a result of decompression. The needle should be left *in situ* until a formal chest drain can be inserted into the midaxillary line (**Figure 1.45**).

INSERTION OF A CHEST DRAIN
- The side of the pneumothorax should be identified.
- A small incision should be made parallel to the ribs in the fourth intercostal in the midaxillary line.
- Blunt dissection using forceps should be carried out until the chest cavity is entered (this may be accompanied by the hiss of escaping air).
- The chest drain should be guided into the thoracic cavity using a pair of artery forceps. Blunt, snub-nosed trocars with spring-loaded tips may be needed to aid entry of the chest tube through the pleura. Sharp-ended or pointed trocars should be avoided (**Figure 1.46**).
- The chest drain should be connected to an underwater seal and the column of water observed to rise and fall with respiration.
- The defect in the skin wall is closed around the tube and the tube secured in place.
- Chest X-ray is taken to confirm the position of the tube.

3. CIRCULATION

MAINTENANCE OF CIRCULATION
A child's blood volume is approximately 75 ml/kg bodyweight. The rate at which this circulates again varies with age. As with breathing rate individual heart rates are of less value than serial measurements.

BLOOD PRESSURE
In childhood, blood pressure changes following fluid loss occur late. The child has an enormous ability to compensate for fluid loss using compensatory mechanisms that maintain flow to vital organs in preference to those that are less vital. Forty to fifty per cent of the circulating blood volume must be lost before blood pressure falls significantly.

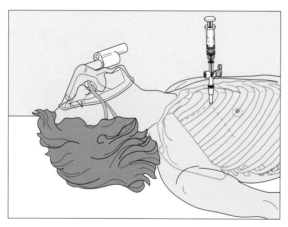

Figure 1.44
Needle thoracotomy. This should be performed by inserting a large-bore needle perpendicular to the skin in the midclavicular line in the second intercostal space. It is helpful to use a needle and cannula, advancing the cannula over the needle once air has been seen to escape. The cannula can then be left in place with minimal further damage to the lung.

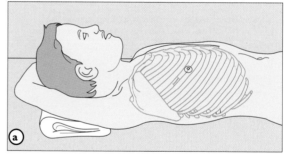

Figure 1.45 a Insertion of a chest drain. The fourth intercostal space is identified in the midaxillary line. An incision parallel to the fourth and fifth ribs is made through the skin and subcutaneous tissue.

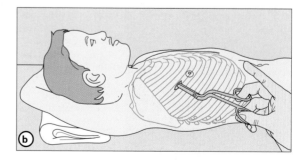

Figure 1.45 b The space is widened using blunt-dissection through the intercostal muscles into the pleural space. A chest drain is then introduced into the thoracic cavity assisted by a pair of artery forceps.

Fluid replacement is dependant on intravenous access which can be difficult in toddlers! A variety of intravenous cannulae are available. **Figure 1.47** shows a selection of cannulae of different sizes made by one manufacturer. It is preferable to become familiar with the use of one type of cannula and to use it consistently unless some over-riding reason prevents this.

As a rule, in emergency medicine, the largest cannula suitable for the size of a child should be used.

Peripheral venous access is usually attempted in the antecubital fossa, (**Figure 1.48**), the back of the hand (**Figure 1.49**), or the saphenous vein (**Figure 1.50**),. These sites are readily accessible, but the chubby infant or toddler can prove difficult even in experienced hands.

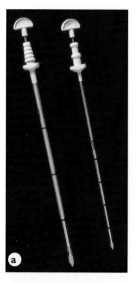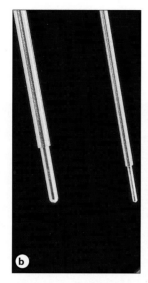

Figure 1.46 a and b
Chest drains with blunt, spring-loaded ends to avoid 'kebab' injury to the intrathoracic organs (see text).

Figure 1.47
A selection of IV cannula from French gauge 22 to French gauge 14.

Figure 1.48
Attempting venous access in the anticubital fossa can often be difficult in toddlers.

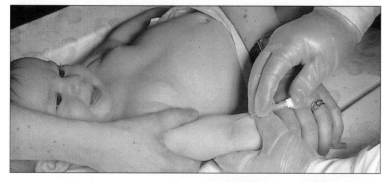

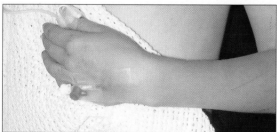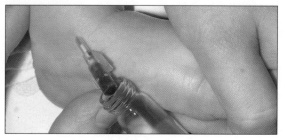

Figure 1.49
An IV cannula in the back of the hand connected to a giving set.

Figure 1.50
IV cannula in a long venous vein with blood being taken from it. Ideally the operator taking blood should be wearing gloves to reduce the chance of cross infection.

Children who have experienced previous repeated cannulation, for example in diabetics, epileptics or children who have spent time in neonatal intensive care, can prove deceptively difficult!

Alternative routes for the insertion of a cannula include the external jugular vein (**Figure 1.51**) and the femoral vein. These should be regarded as peripheral veins initially but subsequently they can be converted to long or central lines using the Seldinger technique (**Figure 1.52**).

Cannulation of the subclavian or jugular veins is difficult in the emergency room (**Figure 1.53**); to be achieved rapidly and effectively it requires an experienced practitioner. However, equipment should be close at hand in case such appropriate expertise is available.

Failure to secure adequate venous access in a child urgently in need of either fluid or drug therapy should prompt the use of the intra-osseous route (**Figure 1.54**).

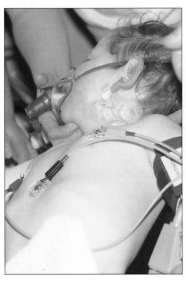

Figure 1.51
The external jugular vein can be cannulated initially and then subsequently converted to a central line using a Seldinger technique.

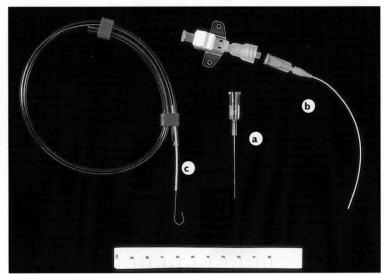

Figure 1.52
Typical central line for use in a small child for monitoring purposes. This will be introduced using a Selinger technique. a = introducer, b = IV lumen, c= Seldinger wire. This narrow gauge long cannula will be a very poor method to transfuse the child should rapid transfusion be needed. It is quite a long tube with a narrow bore and both these factors conspire against rapid transfusion.

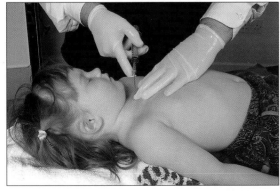

Figure 1.53
Cannulation of the subclavian vein. This is difficult to achieve if other resuscitation procedures are being performed.

- Proximal tibia

- Distal tibia

- Distal femur

Figure 1.54
Suitable sites for intraosseous puncture are listed above.

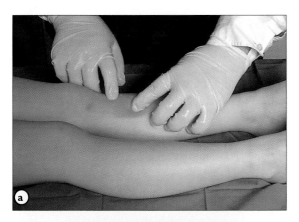

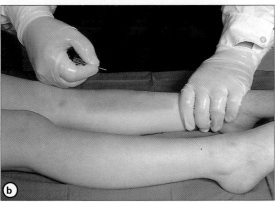

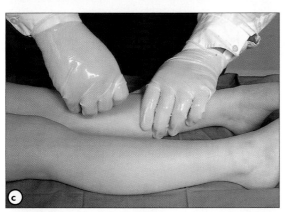

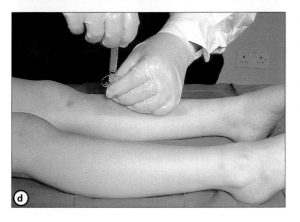

Figure 1.55

a. The proximal tibia has been chosed as a site for insertion of an intraosseous needle. The site has been cleaned with an antiseptic agent

b. The intraosseous needle is held firmly in the hand with the finger and thumb pinching the trochar and cannula approximately 1 cm from the tip.

c. The needle is inserted at the chosen site with a gradual twisting and screwing motion helping downward pressure.

d. The needle has entered the bone and the operator is attempting to aspirate marrow from the marrow cavity.

INTRA-OSSEOUS TECHNIQUE
(Figure 1.55)

- Identify the site to be used.
- Rapidly clean the area with an antiseptic agent.
- Gradually push the intra osseous needle into the bone, with a boring, twisting movement.
- The bone is entered with a give.
- If the needle is in the bone, it will stand proud.
- Connect the tubing and a three-way tap.
- Gently aspirate bone marrow to confirm placement.

All is now ready to infuse drugs or fluids.

Contraindications to intra osseous puncture include:
- Fracture of the bone requiring puncture.
- Burned skin overlying the site.
- Local infection.
- Osteogenesis imperfecta.
- Recent or fresh intra-osseous puncture of the same bone.

Complications of intra-osseous puncture include:
- Fracture if the technique is over-vigorous.
- Epiphyseal damage if too close to the plate.
- Infection if left *in situ* for more than 48 hours.
- Fat embolism.

FLUID THERAPY

Fluid-replacement therapy in children with fluid loss varies from practice to practice. In Europe, colloid solutions are favored, but crystalloid is also used. Our practice is to use normal saline for the first bolus, at a rate of 20 ml/kg rapid-push. Additional resuscitative fluids are administered, as plasma-protein fraction or whole blood in boluses of 10–20 ml/Kg as required, to maintain perfusion.

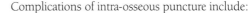

RE-ASSESSMENT

One of the important rules of emergency care is to evaluate every action for effectiveness. Opening the airway should lead to assessment of effectiveness of breathing. If artificial respiration is performed, by either using mouth-to mouth techniques or bag/valve/mask devices, the chest wall must be seent to rise. Similarly, the effect of fluid therapy will be assessed by restoration of peripheral pulses and level of consciousness. These changes will not be instantaneous and take time to come about. Over-aggressive resuscitation, especially with fluid therapy, can be as bad as under-resuscitation. To achieve the correct balance requires training and experience. Junior practitioners should always seek help from senior colleagues if there is doubt or concern about further management of sick children.

'AVPU' scale for assessing level of consciousness

A - Awake

V - Response to **v**erbal stimuli

P - Responds to **p**ainful stimuli

U - **U**nconscious

Figure 1.56

4. DISABILITY

Measurement of disability in young children is very difficult. The ability of a child to understand and comply with the examiner varies considerably. For this reason the Glasgow Coma Score, or its pediatric analogs, can be difficult to apply in a reproducible manner (*see* Chapter 4)

'AVPU' SCALE (Figure 1.56)

The AVPU scale may well be a better screen of altered consciousness in young children and infants than many of the customized pediatric scores. It relies solely on ascertaining whether the child is alert or otherwise, and, if not normal, then attempting to quantify the deficit in a practical manner.

It is important to exclude respiratory or circulatory problems before attributing an altered level of consciousness to an intracerebral lesion.

5. PROGRESS

At this stage an ill or injured child will have been examined, life-threatening problems will have been addressed (at least in part), and some idea of the cause of the illness or injury determined. The needs now are concerned with further stabilization, investigation and transfer. Specialist help should have been sought and a dialog entered into regarding the further management of the child.

Various therapies will be discussed further in the appropriate chapters.

Chapter TWO

Cardiac Arrest

To be presented with a dead or dying child is one of the more distressing areas of clinical practice. Thankfully, cardiac arrest in childhood is extremely rare. Most cases are respiratory in origin, with hypovolemia and shock accounting for most others. Survival is poor once apnea and asystole are evident. Survival rates from full cardiac arrest are poor with resuscitation rates of less than 7% being reported. Even if the child is resuscitated, long-term neurological deficit is common.

Respiratory arrest is preceded by a period of time in which the child experiences increased difficulty in breathing. It is important at this stage to recognize which children are at risk and to take remedial action before the arrest occurs. The same applies to hypovolemia and shock. However, if the child has gone into cardiac arrest, it is imperative that a controlled, well organized approach to the resuscitation attempt is made in order for the child to have any chance of recovery.

Most recommendations for the treatment of cardiac arrest are consensus views only and are based on the current understanding of the underlying causes and the potential benefits of the treatments available. These approaches to treatment are open to review and will be revised with time, hopefully following critical analysis of the available evidence.

Bearing this in mind, three distinct progressions in cardiac arrest management can be defined. These are:
- Basic life support.
- Intermediate life support.
- Advanced life support.

BASIC LIFE SUPPORT

Basic life support is a skill which should be learned by all members of the population both lay and medical. It involves:
- Recognition of the arrested child.
- The ability to open an airway and establish ventilation.
- The ability to maintain circulation.

For the purpose of simplicity, children are divided into two groups:
- Those under 12 months of age.
- Those over 12 months of age.

Resuscitation in the new-born period has been excluded although the principles are the same.

Again, for the purposes of simplicity, it is taken that adolescence and the onset of puberty are indicative of the upper-age limit for categorizing an individual as a child.

As discussed in chapter 1 the heart occupies a different position in infants than older children and requires different hand placings for cardiac massage. Apart from this the techniques and principles of resuscitation are similar in both age groups.

RECOGNITION OF CARDIAC ARREST

Cardiac arrest is defined as the cessation of respiration and an absence of cardiac output; both result in loss of consciousness. The first step, therefore, is to establish that coma is indeed present and that the child is not asleep. This should be done by gently shaking or stimulating the child (**Figures 2.1 a and 2.2 a**). If the child fails to respond then coma can be said to be present. The child is immediately at risk of asphyxia through loss of reflexes. This loss of reflexes results in the tongue falling back into the pharynx with consequent respiratory obstruction. Similarly, loss of gag reflexes will allow vomit and regurgitated food to enter the airway.

AIRWAY

The next step is to secure the airway as best one can. This is achieved by the simple chin lift/ head-tilt maneuver. The chin is lifted by placing the hand on the mandible and bringing the jaw upwards and forwards. Occasionally, the jaw will need to be thrust forward by pressure on the angles of the mandible. At the same time the head should be tilted gently until it is in the so-called sniffing position (**Figures 2.1 b and 2.2 b**).

The mouth should be opened and briefly examined. Any **obvious** foreign body should be removed. Once the head is in this position the patency of the airway can be assessed by looking, listening and feeling for air movement (**Figures 2.1 c and 2.2 c**).

BREATHING

Simple measures, such as opening the airway, may be all that is required to establish a normal breathing pattern. If breathing is absent, gasping, or otherwise ineffective, artificial ventilation should be instituted. In small infants it may be possible to cover the mouth and nose with the rescuer's mouth. This should be done where possible. In older children it may only be possible to cover mouth or nose (**Figures 2.1 d and 2.2 d**).

Five steady breaths are then given taking time to take in a fresh breath between each. Each rescue breath should be sufficient to cause the chest wall to rise.

CIRCULATION

Once artificial ventilation has been started the circulation has to be assessed. This is best done by feeling for a major pulse. In the infant this can be achieved by either feeling the femoral or brachial pulse (**Figure 2.1 e**). In older children the carotid may be more convenient (**Figure 2.2 e**). If the pulse is absent, or it is less than 60 beats per minute in infants, external cardiac massage must be commenced.

EXTERNAL CARDIAC MASSAGE TECHNIQUE
Infants

Two methods of cardiac compression are available in infants. These include:

1. Using the index finger and middle finger on the sternum one finger breadth below the internipple line (**Figure 2.1 f**).
2. Using two thumbs over the same point as above with the rest of the hands encircling the chest.

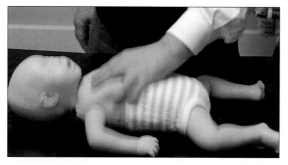

Figure 2.1 a
Assessment of level of consciousness in an infant. The child is gently shaken and stimulated.

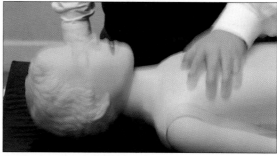

Figure 2.2 a
Assessment of level of consciousness in an older child. The child is gently shaken and stimulated.

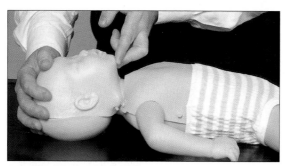

Figure 2.1 b
Chin lift/head tilt. One hand is placed on the child's forehead while the other hand gently lifts the mandible forward taking care not to hold any of the soft tissues behind the mandible.

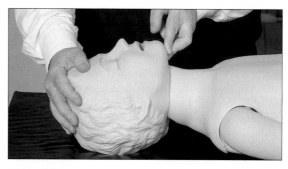

Figure 2.2 b
Chin lift/head tilt. The head is steadied by placing one hand on the forehead while one hand grasps the mandible and brings it forward.

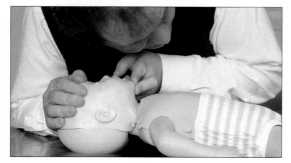

Figure 2.1 c
Look, listen and feel for any air entry. Supporting the chin and forehead, feel for air on the side of the face, listen for air entry and watch for chest wall movement now that the airway is opened.

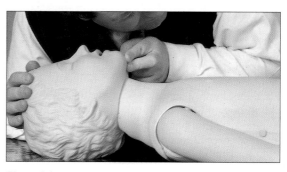

Figure 2.2 c
Having supported the chin and forehead, feel for air on the side of the face and both listen for air entry and watch for movement of the chest wall. Look, listen and feel for any air entry.

Method 2 is probably slightly more effective but can be very difficult to achieve in single-person resuscitation. It is therefore recommended only if two or more people are present at the resuscitation; otherwise method 1 should be used.

In older children the heel of the hand is placed over the lower-third of the sternum (**Figure 2.2 f**).

The rate of compression should be equivalent to 100 beats per minute. A total of five compressions should be performed. One should then return to ventilating the child by mouth and give one breath as described above.

RESUSCITATION CYCLE

Once artificial ventilation and cardiac compression have been started they should be continued at a ratio of five compressions to 1 breath. This should be done over a period of approximately one minute. At this stage the child should be

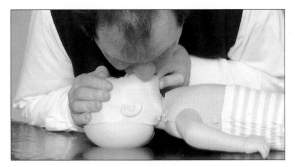

Figure 2.1 d
Artificial ventilation. The rescuer covers the infant's mouth and nose with his mouth and delivers five steady breaths, each time watching the chest wall rise.

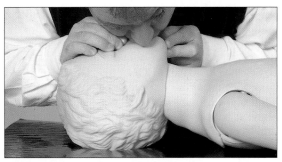

Figure 2.2 d
The rescuer covers the child's mouth with his mouth and delivers five steady breaths, each time watching the chest wall rise.

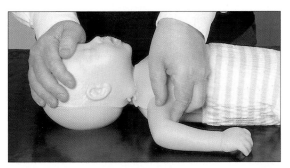

Figure 2.1 e
Assess circulation. In an infant this is achieved by feeling the brachial pulse between the elbow and the axilla.

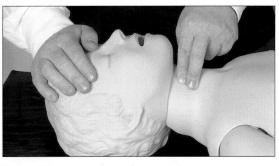

Figure 2.2 e
Assess circulation. In an older child this is best done by palpating the carotid area lateral to the thyroid cartilage and medial to the sternocleidomastoid muscle.

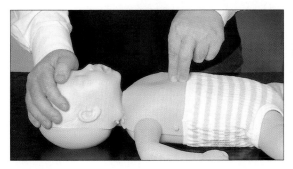

Figure 2.1 f
Cardiac compression in an infant. Two fingers are placed one finger-breadth below the internipple line over the sternum. Downward compressions are applied using two fingers.

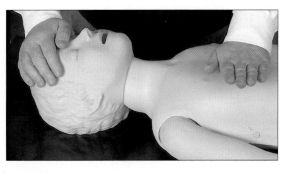

Figure 2.2 f
Cardiac compression in an older child. The heel of the hand is placed on the lower-third of the sternum and downward compressions are applied using a straight arm.

re-assessed. If there is still no return of spontaneous circulation or respiration the rescuer must seek help from elsewhere.

This will involve calling an ambulance and trained personnel to the scene. If the child is already at the hospital, the resuscitation team should be called.

Once extra help has been summoned, the rescuer should return to basic life-support measures which should be continued at a rate of five compressions to 1 ventilation stopping every 10 cycles to re-assess circulation and respiration (**Figure 2.3**).

If the child regains a pulse and begins breathing spontaneously, he or she should be placed in the recovery position (**Figure 2.4**).

STOPPING RESUSCITATION

Basic life support will be practiced by lay people in the main and without any adjuncts. Resuscitation should not therefore be stopped until either trained medical help has arrived or the rescuer is exhausted.

INTERMEDIATE LIFE SUPPORT

This has often been described as basic life support with adjuncts. All medically trained people and nursing staff should be able to perform intermediate life support effectively:

- The first available adjunct is the oropharyngeal airway. If there is difficulty in maintaining an airway a suitably sized oropharyngeal airway should be inserted. This may help maintain the patency of the airway and make ventilation easier (**Figure 2.5**, *see* **also Figure 1.31**).
- The second adjunct is suction (**Figure 2.6**, *see* **also Figure 1.30**). Rigid Yankauer suction catheters are best. Flexible catheters may be used to suck secretions from endotracheal tubes.
- The third adjunct is the delivery of high-concentration oxygen, using positive-pressure ventilation, through a bag/valve/mask device.

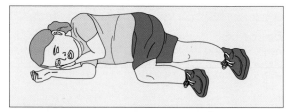

Figure 2.4
Recovery position. The recovery position will help to protect the airway in an unconscious child who has regained a pulse and respiration.

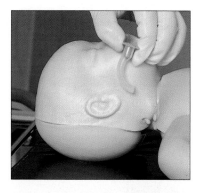

Figure 2.5
Sizing a Guedal airway. The correct size can be determined by placing the Guedal airway to the side of the child's head. The correctly sized airway should extend from the angle of the mouth to the angle of the jaw.

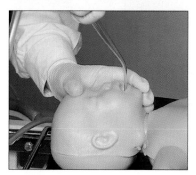

Figure 2.6
Secretions can be gently removed by using a rigid Yankauer sucker.

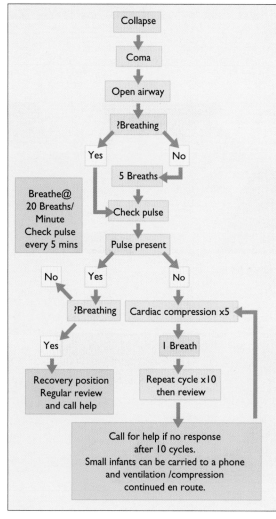

Figure 2.3
Flow chart for Basic Life Support.

Several different methods for oxygen delivery exist. These include:
- A bag-valve-mask device (**Figure 1.42**).
- A pediatric anesthetic circuit (**Figure 1.43**).

Both rely on delivering oxygen through a well fitting mask, either round or triangular. Correct application of the mask and the ability to open the airway at the same time take training and considerable skill (**Figure 2.7**).

Some practitioners are unable to maintain an airway with one hand and therefore a two-handed technique is preferable. In this situation a second operator should be available to deliver the oxygen.

The choice between a self-inflating bag and an anesthetic circuit is personal. There is no doubt that the self-inflating bag is easier to use for personnel untrained in administrating anesthetics. However, because anesthetists are frequently called to the resuscitation room, both types of equipment should be available.

OTHER ADJUNCTS

In many situations it will be possible to determine the underlying rhythm associated with the cardiac arrest by connecting an electrocardiogram (ECG) monitor to the child's chest. While many staff may not have the knowledge or authority to deliver further treatment they should certainly be in a position to present more experienced staff with a working diagnosis, e.g. a diagnosis of the current rhythm.

ADVANCED LIFE SUPPORT

Advanced life support involves:
- The ability to establish a definitive airway.
- The ability to establish intravenous access.
- The ability to recognize underlying rhythms from the electrocardiogram.
- The ability to correctly treat each of these rhythms according to protocols.
- The ability to decide when to terminate resuscitation.

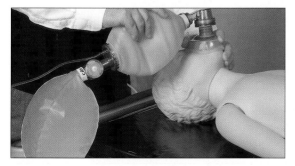

Figure 2.7
Bag-valve-mask ventilation. The left hand holds the mask closely against the face at the same time lifting the mandible forward. The right hand compresses the bag. On each compression of the bag, the chest wall should be seen to rise.

DEFINITIVE AIRWAY CARE

Definitive airway care involves the insertion of an endotracheal tube, either orally or nasally, and the ability to create a surgical airway.

ENDOTRACHEAL INTUBATION (*see* Chapter 1)

Before any attempt is made to intubate a child adequate oxygenation must have taken place using a bag-valve-mask device. Also the operator must be skilled in intubation and must take no more than 45 seconds to achieve intubation.

INTRAVENOUS ACCESS

Peripheral venous access is usually easiest and safest to achieve. Failure to establish intravenous access within 90 seconds in a child in cardiac arrest should lead one to perform intra osseous puncture. Acceptable alternative sites for cannulation are the femoral vein and external jugular vein. There is little place for direct central-venous puncture in a cardiac arrest situation; it is not very practical to perform cardiac massage while the procedure is carried out and stopping cardiac massage is not desirable.

All of these procedures have been described previously (*see* Chapter 1).

RECOGNITION OF UNDERLYING ARRHYTHMIA

By the time advanced life support measures are considered, an ECG monitor should be connected to the child. In a cardiac arrest situation, one of three underlying rhythms needs to be considered:
- Asystole.
- Ventricular fibrillation.
- Electromechanical dissociation.

These are often termed 'collapse' rhythms.

ASYSTOLE (Figure 2.8 and 2.12)

Asystole is the most common collapse rhythm found in childhood. It is characterized by a flat trace on the electrocardiograph. Before it can be diagnosed the following checks should be carried out:
- That the machine is not in 'paddles' mode.
- That the leads are actually connected to the patient.
- That the gain is turned up to maximum.

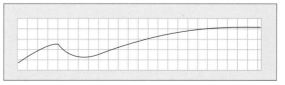

Figure 2.8
Asystole. The gain should be turned up to maximum to ensure that ventriculation fibrillation is not the cause.

With regard to the latter point when the gain is turned up to maximum a very fine fluctuation compatible with ventricular fibrillation may be identified. In this situation it is probably better to treat the child as if in ventricular fibrillation and follow this algorithm. (**Figure 2.9** and **2.12**)

VENTRICULAR FIBRILLATION (Figure 2.9 and 2.12)

Ventricular fibrillation is characterized by chaotic patterns on the ECG recording. Traditionally, it is defined as either coarse or fine although the implications for each are not really clear.

Hypothermia, electric shock and drug overdose predispose to ventricular fibrillation.

Ventricular tachycardia is rare in children (**Figure 2.10**) and is usually due to drug intoxication or hypoxia. If unstable it should be treated as ventricular fibrillation (*see* above). If stable, it must be differentiated from supraventricular tachycardia and treated accordingly (*see* Cardiac Problems)

ELECTROMECHANICAL DISSOCIATION (EMD) (Figure 2.11 and 2.12)

This may better be described as pulseless electrical activity (PEA). The ECG demonstrates QRS complex often at a very slow rate. No pulse is palpable although an impulse wave may be seen from an indwelling artery catheter. If this is present the blood pressure usually goes no higher than 10–20 mm Hg.

Electromechanical dissociation may be associated with tension pneumothorax, hypovolemia, hyperkalemia and other electrolyte disturbances.

DRUG AND TREATMENT PROTOCOLS

The treatment for each of the above arrhythmias is considered on the accompanying flow chart (**Figure 2.12**).

STOPPING RESUSCITATION

The decision to stop resuscitation is a very difficult one. Many factors need to be considered and the interplay between these is considerable.

The decision to stop resuscitation is never easy but is one that must be made with the fullest information possible.

A critical review of progress at 30 minutes is advisable. In the absence of hypothermia, submersion, or poisoning there may well be little point in progressing. However, no two situations are identical and each should be judged on its merits.

IMMERSION INJURY

Immersion injury can lead to **drowning** (death following immersion) or **near-drowning** (survival).

In some parts of the world, drowning and near-drowning are common problems. The British climate and the lack of domestic swimming pools makes drowning a relatively rare event in that country.

The principles of resuscitating a child who has been immersed are identical to those detailed above. Factors that affect the success of the resuscitation include:
- Length of time immersed.
- Temperature of the water.
- Time to resuscitation.

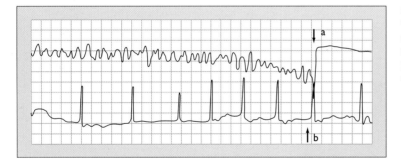

Figure 2.9
Ventricular fibrillation. D C shock has been applied at 'a'. After a brief period of asystole QRS complexes reappeared and a pulse became palpable at the carotid artery marked 'b'.

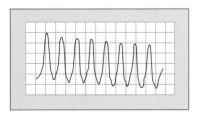

Figure 2.10
Ventricular tachycardia.

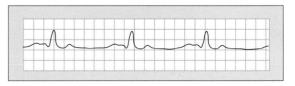

Figure 2.11
Electromechanical dissociation. QRS complexes associated with no pulse (pulseless electrical activity (PEA)) are present.

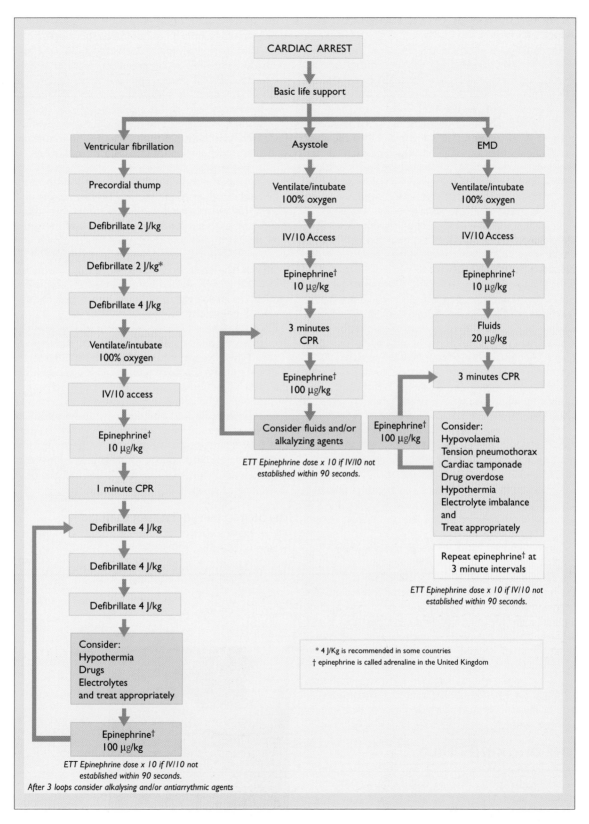

Figure 2.12
Algorithm for treatment of 'collapse rhythms' found in cardiac arrest.

IMMERSION-ASSOCIATED CARDIAC ARREST

Children who are in cardiac arrest following immersion should be resuscitated using the procedures detailed above. Care must be taken to protect the cervical spine if a diving injury is suspected, as cervical spine injury is likely (*see* Trauma chapter, **Figure 4.3**).

The core temperature should be measured as soon as possible. If the temperature is low (<34.5ºC) the child should be warmed by whatever means possible. At the very least, further heat loss should be avoided by wrapping the child in blankets and getting him or her to a warm, dry environment. Resuscitation should be continued until the child has reached normal body temperature. Defibrillation and drug therapy are not effective when core temperatures are below 32ºC.

NEAR-DROWNING

If the child is gasping or has a pulse after immersion, respiratory and circulatory support will be necessary; 100% oxygen should be given as soon as possible. Ventilatory support using a bag/valve/mask device should be used. Aspiration of water leads to loss of surfactant with subsequent development of respiratory distress syndrome. This may be complicated by pulmonary edema, which can develop any time in the 24 hours after immersion. Ventilatory support using positive end expiratory pressure (PEEP) is often required.

Circulatory collapse is common following near-drowning. Fluid replacement and inotropic support should be considered and all fluid should be given warmed if possible.

Blood gases should be assessed as early as possible. They may give the first clue as to the development of respiratory compromise, respiratory distress (falling O_2 and rising CO_2) or both.

A chest X-ray is mandatory, as is a cervical spine film if diving cannot be ruled out. Full spinal cord protection should be maintained until the spine is cleared.

Antibiotics should be administered if the child has been immersed in dirty water or sewerage (slurry pit); they should be effective against coliforms and anaerobes as well as Gram-positive organisms. If open wounds are present, tetanus status should be determined and treated accordingly (*see* Wound Care, **Figure 4.139**).

All children who suffer near-drowning should be admitted for a period of observation. Those in need of resuscitation should go to a high-dependency area or intensive care setting.

THE CHOKING CHILD

Airway obstruction, due to a foreign body, is not an infrequent cause of death in childhood. Young children are more at risk than older children.

It is difficult to distinguish partial airway obstruction from a foreign body in the esophagus as both can present with stridor and drooling. Any child who is alert and awake should be brought to hospital as soon as possible. Once in the emergency room the child should be assessed as rapidly as possible and arrangements made to remove the foreign body in a safe, controlled environment. The child should stay in the resuscitation room until transfer can be arranged.

Children with foreign bodies in the esophagus may be amenable to having the foreign body removed by an experienced radiologist (*see* **Figures 5.21 and 5.22**).

Complete airway obstruction is a catastrophic event. The child is seen to be making respiratory effort to no avail. and rapidly becomes cyanosed before lapsing into a coma. In this situation it is important to act with speed. Any infant suspected of having a complete airway obstruction should immediately be turned upside down and slapped five times vigorously on the back (**Figure 2.13**). With luck, the foreign body will be ejected into the mouth and possibly even ejected from the mouth completely. Normal respiration will be resumed immediately and the child will be perfectly safe.

If the child has lapsed into a coma and back blows have failed, the child should be placed in the supine position and given five chest thrusts (**Figure 2.14**). After these, the child's mouth should be opened and any foreign body removed. If the foreign body is not readily visible, five breaths should be administered. This procedure should follow the same technique outlined for airway control in the section above on basic life support. This should then be followed by five back blows, five chest thrusts and further ventilatory efforts. It is prudent to continue this sequence until either help arrives or the child has been asystolic for a considerable period of time.

CHOKING IN THE OLDER CHILD

Older children may be more difficult to up-end. If they are struggling to make respiratory effort, back blows may be helpful in removing the foreign body. The Heimlich maneuver may also be appropriate (**Figure 2.15**)

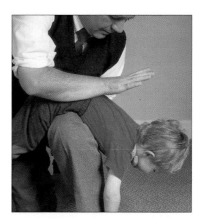

Figure 2.13
Back blows in an infant will often dislodge a foreign body in the airway.

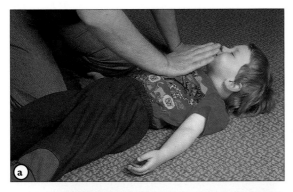

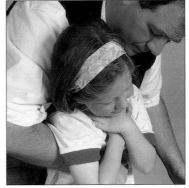

Figure 2.15
The Heimlich maneuver. This is useful in older children.

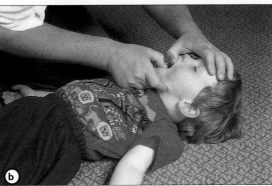

Figure 2.14 a and b
(a) Chest thrusts. These may be needed in the unconscious child if back blows are unsuccessful at clearing an obstruction. (b) Always check the mouth after each procedure to ensure the foreign body is not in the pharynx.

If the child lapses into a coma, back blows should be followed by chest thrusts. These should in turn be followed by ventilatory effort as above. The next cycle should consist of back blows and abdominal thrusts. This again should be followed by ventilation. This cycle should be continued until either the foreign body is removed or the child has been asystolic for a considerable length of time.

ORGANIZATION OF CARDIAC ARREST
(Figure 2.16)

A well organized resuscitation is much more effective than one in which panic and lack of communication prevail. There are many ways to organize cardiac arrest treatment.

It is important that everyone understands their role and that a senior and experienced doctor takes absolute control of the resuscitation procedure (Doctor 1). He or she should remain at the head end of the patient and direct all aspects of the procedure in treating the child. This doctor has overall responsibility for the care of the child as well as airway control. The practical procedures and protocols should be called out as required and, ideally, this doctor's voice should be the only one heard in the resuscitation room.

Doctor 2 should perform cardiac massage. If insufficient doctors are available this role can be taken by anyone

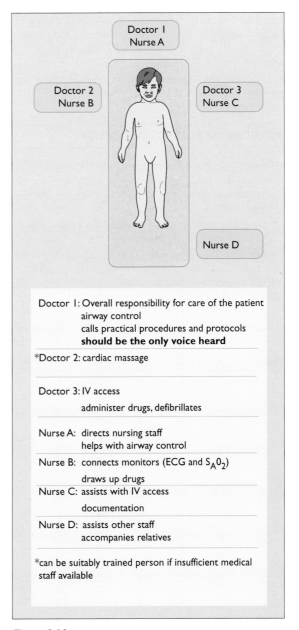

Doctor 1
Nurse A

Doctor 2
Nurse B

Doctor 3
Nurse C

Nurse D

Doctor 1: Overall responsibility for care of the patient
airway control
calls practical procedures and protocols
should be the only voice heard

*Doctor 2: cardiac massage

Doctor 3: IV access
administer drugs, defibrillates

Nurse A: directs nursing staff
helps with airway control

Nurse B: connects monitors (ECG and S_AO_2)
draws up drugs

Nurse C: assists with IV access
documentation

Nurse D: assists other staff
accompanies relatives

*can be suitably trained person if insufficient medical staff available

Figure 2.16

who is able to do cardiac massage. It is important that Doctor 1 supervises the cardiac massage technique.

Doctor 3 has the initial role of trying to establish intravenous access. If a peripheral vein is not cannulated within 90 seconds or three attempts (whichever is the later), intraosseous access should be obtained. This should then be used to administer all drugs and resuscitation fluids. If defibrillation is required this doctor should perform the task.

The nurses should also organize themselves into a smooth functioning team. A minimum of four nurses are required and their roles are given below. It is important that Nurse A is a senior and experienced member of the nursing staff who is fully conversant with airway care. Nurses B and C should work together to help establish intravenous access and to ensure that the patient is monitored. Drawing up drugs is a difficult and time-consuming task and requires more than one nurse at times. Nurse D should help where required but should pay particular attention to the relatives to make sure that they are looked after. A system for documenting treatment as it is administered is important. This helps in future audit and analysis.

POSTRESUSCITATION CARE

Following successful resuscitation of a child from cardiac arrest one should immediately arrange to transfer the child to the intensive care unit. Almost certainly the child will be intubated and active ventilation will be in progress. Often intubation and ventilation will have been achieved without any paralysis or sedation. As the effectiveness of spontaneous circulation delivers oxygenated blood to the brain the child may become agitated. Consideration should now be given to formal sedation and paralysis of the child to allow ventilation to continue.

It is imperative to secure an endotracheal tube and to ensure that ventilation is equal in both lung fields. Central lines should be inserted and their position should be checked by chest X-ray. Once the position is confirmed to be accurate, the lines should be firmly secured in place to avoid them being removed during transfer. These lines will facilitate monitoring and inotropic support.

Consideration should also be given to inserting a nasogastric tube to decompress the stomach.

All documentation should be completed, particularly with reference to the therapy that has been instituted to secure the successful survival of the child. All blood test results that are available, together with ECG recordings and X-rays, and any other clinical information should be gathered together and transferred with the child to the intensive care unit.

En route the child should be monitored using whatever means are available. Ideally, this should include a cardiac monitor and a pulse oximeter. The child should be accompanied to the intensive-care unit by the most senior medical and nursing staff available. They should be able to continue full airway care and also be accompanied by sufficient drugs to maintain sedation and re-institute cardiac arrest procedures should the child re-arrest on the way to the unit.

POSTRESUSCITATION PROCEDURES

The resuscitation room should be immediately restocked, replacing all equipment that has been used in order to be prepared for the next child.

If the child has died, it is important to inform his or her GP, health visitor and the legal authorities as soon as possible.

COUNSELING

It is important to have a debrief for staff a few days after the death of a child within the AED. This will allow staff to discuss the resuscitation and its effectiveness; it will also help them to come to terms with the grief reaction.

Chapter THREE

The Child and Medical Emergencies

Medical emergencies are frequent and numerous in the Accident and Emergency Department (AED). They affect children of all ages. However, respiratory emergencies are particularly common during the winter months and affect younger children more than they do older children. For the purposes of this section, medical emergencies will be broadly grouped into the following categories:

- Respiratory disease.
- Neurologic disease.
- Cardiac disease.
- Renal disorders.
- Diabetic problems.
- Anaphylaxis/allergic reactions.
- Gastroenteritis.
- Acute poisoning.
- Hematology.
- Unwell child.
- Dermatologic manifestations of systemic disease.
- Sepsis.

RESPIRATORY DISEASE

Respiratory admissions account for significant numbers of medical attendances and admissions throughout the winter months. Common conditions include:

- Asthma.
- Bronchiolitis.
- Croup/stridor.
- Pneumonia.

The role of the AED in managing these patients is (a) to identify those children who require inpatient treatment as distinct from those who can be discharged and sent home and (b) to provide appropriate care to all. Many factors play a part in these decisions, not least the ability of the parents to cope and the general social conditions at home (**Figure 3.1**)

Children with chronic respiratory disease, for example, cystic fibrosis or bronchopulmonary dysplasia are at particular risk from the effects of bronchiolitis and these children should be treated with circumspection. If in doubt, management of these children should be discussed with their long-term chest physician.

ASTHMA

Asthma is defined as reversible airway disease. It is precipitated by many causes including viral infection, contact with allergens, exercise or cold. Cold- and virally-induced asthma are more common during the winter months than in the summer. The other causes have to be considered throughout the year.

PRESENTATION

Children can be grouped into one of four broad categories determined by the severity of the presenting symptoms. The symptoms and signs that are associated with these categories are summarized (**Figure 3.2**).

Life-Threatening Asthma

It can be difficult to distinguish between severe and life-threatening asthma in the emergency situation. Both are associated with rapid respiratory rates and reduced peak expiratory flow rate (PEFR). It may be impossible to obtain a PEFR in children, but proxies for this include the ability to talk and a history of their recent feeding.

If possible, peak flow measurements should be attempted (**Figure 3.3**). Most children over the age of four can make an attempt at using a peak flow meter. The peak flow should be expressed as a percentage of the predicted value for that child or as a percentage of the best peak flow recorded.

With regard to talking, children in severe distress may only be able to manage two or three words in a sentence without having to gasp for breath. Those with life-threatening asthma may not be able to speak at all. For the same reason, i.e. severe respiratory distress, their ability to eat is substantially reduced.

Clinical indications that a child with respiratory disease may need to be admitted

1. Exhaustion – manifests by increased respiratory effort and increasing inability to cope.
2. Failure to respond to treatment in the AED
3. Decreased feeding despite treatment
4. A toxic child
5. Poor social circumstances

Figure 3.1

A rapid pulse rate (>140 beats per minute) and a decreasing level of consciousness are both significant signs of severe disease; the latter is a sign of hypoxia. With regard to other features, wheezing will be apparent in mild, moderate and severe cases of asthma. The quality or the distribution of the wheeze is of little help in making the diagnosis.

The development of a quiet chest is a very sinister feature and one which suggests that collapse is imminent. This sign is of particular importance.

The child should be triaged immediately to the resuscitation room with a brief assessment as detailed above. While this is going on, 100% oxygen should be administered and intravenous access obtained. A β_2-agonist (salbutamol or terbutaline) can be administered via a nebulizer as soon as it can be obtained (**Figure 3.4**).

If the child has not had previous theophylline treatment, a loading dose of intravenous aminophylline 5 mg/kg over 20 minutes under electrocardiographic control, followed by a maintenance infusion of 1 mg/kg/hour should be administered. If the child has already been on oral theophylline, the loading dose should be omitted.

Intravenous hydrocortisone should be administered at a dose of 100 mg 6-hourly. The child may be moderately dehydrated due to lack of fluid intake; daily fluid requirements should be given intravenously if this is the case. This is particularly important if the child is unable to drink adequately.

It is important not to delay treatment in these children. It takes time to calculate the dose requirements of the child and to draw up the correct doses of aminophylline and hydrocortisone. For this reason nebulized salbutamol is indicated as soon as the child presents.

The child should be transferred as soon as possible to an intensive care unit and monitored closely during the transfer period. Heart, respiratory rate, PEFR and oxygen saturation should all be monitored until the child reaches the intensive care unit.

Blood gas analysis may be helpful adjunct to clinical assessment it is helpful in charting progress and determining the need for artificial ventilation. A rising partial pressure of carbon dioxide and falling partial pressure of oxygen are harbingers of respiratory failure.

Multiple arterial puncture is undesirable in children. If repeated analysis of blood gases is deemed necessary an indwelling arterial catheter should be used.

Severe asthma

The child should be triaged to the resuscitation room and assessed as above. High-flow oxygen should be given via a face mask while waiting for a β_2-agonist to be prepared.

	Mild asthma	Moderate asthma	Severe asthma	Life-threatening asthma
Respiratory rate	Normal or mildly raised	Raised	>50	>50
*Peak expiratory flow rate (PEFR)	>75% expected value	50–75% expected value	33–50% expected value	<33% expected value
Ability to talk	Normal	Normal or reduced	Poor	No
Heart rate	Normal or mildly raised	Raised	>140	>140 *or slowing heart (beware)*
Level of consciousness	Normal	Normal	Drowsy/ confused	Reduced/coma
Other features	Wheeze	Wheeze	Wheeze	Quiet chest *(beware)*

* Not all children are able to perform PEFR, especially if in respiratory distress.

Figure 3.2

The drug should be delivered via a nebulizer driven by oxygen. Steroid, in the form of prednisolone, 2 mg/kg bodyweight to a maximum of 40 mg, should be given orally. There is a good case for giving intravenous hydrocortisone as for life-threatening asthma.

Oxygen saturation and heart rate should be monitored to detect changes suggestive of deterioration (**Figure 3.5**).

The child should be assessed regularly. If the child has deteriorated, despite treatment, a new regime appropriate to the treatment of life-threatening asthma should be initiated. If the child stays the same, or is improving, β_2-agonist nebulizers can be given every 30 minutes. Again, the child should be admitted to a high-dependency area as soon as possible.

Moderate asthma

The child with moderate asthma should be triaged into an urgent category but does not necessarily need to be kept in the resuscitation room. The child should be given nebullized β_2-agonists and oral prednisolone 2 mg/kg (to a maximum 40 mg). The child should be re-assessed after 15 minutes and a further assessment made.

If the condition is deteriorating, a decision should be made to admit the child for further inpatient treatment. Another β_2-agonist administered via a nebulizer can be given while this is being arranged.

If the child is showing some improvement, further β_2-agonists administered via a nebulizer may be given in the emergency room (maximum of two) with the child being

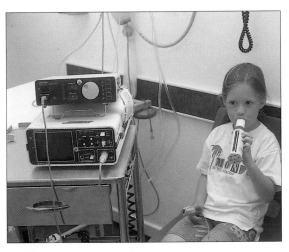

Figure 3.3
Peak flow should be measured, if at all possible, in children with asthma.

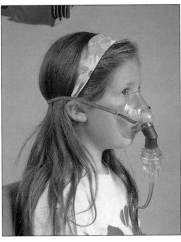

Figure 3.4
A child receiving nebulized salbutamol through a mask. Wherever possible the device should be driven by oxygen.

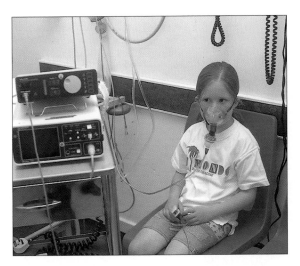

Figure 3.5
All children with severe airway disease should be monitored. In this situation a heart monitor and pulse oximeter are being used.

re-assessed after each. If the child has improved considerably, and the parents are happy and home circumstances permit, the child may be allowed home to be followed up by their doctor.

Prior to discharge the doctor should ensure that the child has adequate β₂-agonist and steroid inhalers to continue treatment at home, and that the child is able to operate his or her inhaler proficiently (**Figure 3.6**). It should also be ensured that the parents of the child are able to come back to the emergency room should there be any deterioration in his or her condition. A further 4-days' supply of prednisolone 2 mg/kg should be provided. If these criteria cannot be met, the child should be admitted.

Mild asthma

Children often present to the AED with mild asthma. However, the presentation is often atypical. Children can present with persistent cough or repeated antibiotic usage for 'chest infections'. In these situations, asthma should be excluded and a trial of prophylactic treatment, for example, sodium cromoglycate or steroid inhaler, offered.

Mild asthma can usually be well managed by family doctors in the community. A discussion of the treatment regime is beyond the scope of this text.

If exercise-induced asthma is apparent, use of a β-agonist inhaler prior to exercise may be all that is needed.

CHEST RADIOGRAPHY IN ACUTE ASTHMA
(Figures 3.7 and 3.8)

Chest X-ray is seldom indicated in acute asthma. Factors that may influence the decision to carry out a chest X-ray are:

- First asthmatic attack (but not neccesarily as an emergency).
- Failure to respond to treatment.
- Clinical evidence of infection or pneumothorax.

BRONCHIOLITIS

Bronchiolitis is a seasonal illness occurring predominantly in the winter months. It typically affects children less than 18 months of age.

Usually, a child presents with a history of upper respiratory tract infection followed by gradual onset of wheeze and increasing respiratory effort. Physical signs include:

- Tachypnea.
- Tachycardia.
- Scattered wheeze.
- Scattered crepitations.
- Liver edge more than 1 cm below the costal margin.

Many children with this illness can be managed at home. Admission to hospital, however, should be arranged if the child is deteriorating; symptoms suggestive of deterioration are increased respiratory effort, poor feeding or the development of signs compatible with pneumonia. Apnoeic attacks or episodes are an absolute indication to admit.

No single treatment exists for this disorder in the AED. Nebulized ipratropium bromide may help dry secretions and consequently make respiratory distress slightly less pronounced. The effect, however, soon wears off and repeat doses may be necessary. It may, however, buy time to enable the child to feed and to regain some strength. β-agonists have not been shown to have any real benefit in this condition unless wheeze predominates. Sitting semi-recumbent

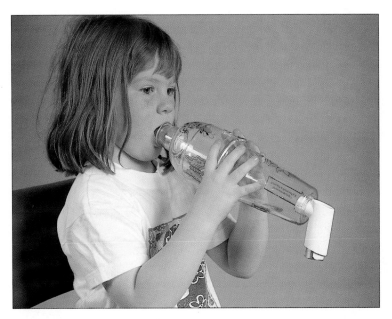

Figure 3.6
This child was not getting any benefit from her inhaled β-agonist. When her technique was checked it was found that the metered-dose inhaler was being inserted upside down. Once this was corrected a dramatic improvement in her symptoms was noted.

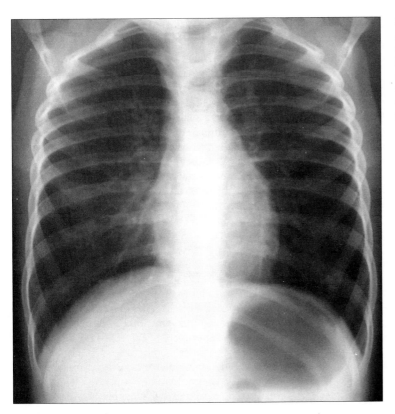

Figure 3.7
Anteroposterior chest X-ray of a child with an acute asthmatic attack. This reveals bilateral overinflation of the lung fields, central peribronchial thickening and right middle-lobe consolidation revealed by loss of the sharp outline of the right cardiac margin.

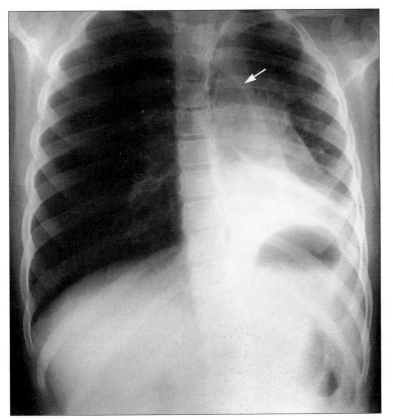

Figure 3.8
Posteroanterior chest X-ray of a child with acute asthma. This demonstrates a consolidated collapsed left lower lobe identified by the triangular opacity behind the heart. Note the small left hemithorax compensatory expansion of the right lung with herniation across the midline. Pleural reflection is arrowed. The obstruction of the left lower lobe was caused by a mucous plug.

and mist therapy may also help. Most children with bronchiolitis can be managed at home, but some will require admission (*see* **Figure 3.1**).

Antibiotics are not indicated in the initial treatment of bronchiolitis. Indeed, they may add complications such as diarrhea and vomiting which will worsen symptoms. Therefore, antibiotics must be used judiciously, if at all.

The signs and symptoms classifying respiratory distress are similar to asthma. If a child is allowed home, the following general principles should be followed:

- The child should be kept propped up as much as possible. This may be facilitated by nursing the child in a car seat.
- Regular small feeds should be given which will help keep the child nourished.
- Exposure to moisture may help in relieving symptoms.
- Parents should be advised to return or seek further medical advice if they are unhappy with the child at any stage.

CROUP/STRIDOR

Stridor is a condition whereby there is noisy inspiration associated with partial upper airway obstruction. Causes include:

- Epiglottitis.
- Croup (laryngotracheobronchitis).
- Inhaled foreign bodies.

Figure 3.9 shows the clinical pictures associated with the three diagnoses.

EPIGLOTTITIS

Epiglottitis is a potentially life-threatening illness typically caused by *Haemophilus influenzae* type B. Recent programs to immunize young children against this pathogen will hopefully reduce the incidence of the illness over a period of time.

Epiglottitis is basically a clinical diagnosis. It is important to establish guidelines for managing epiglottitis prior to the child arriving at the AED.

The general principles of care are as follows:

- Keep the child in as comfortable a position as possible, even if this means leaving the child on his or her mother's knee.
- **Do not interfere with the child in any way. This especially means not attempting to look into the throat. Other interventions, such as applying a nebulizer, can also be harmful.**
- No attempts should be made at intravenous access as this may also stimulate complete airway obstruction.
- X-rays are of no proven help as the diagnosis is a clinical one and X-rays will not alter the management (**Figure 3.10**).
- The child should be kept in a resuscitation room with full resuscitation equipment available. Only when everything is fully prepared should attempts be made to induce anesthesia and intubate the child; these procedures have to be conducted in a controlled manner.

Ideally, intubation should be carried out in theatre with facilities available to perform either a tracheotomy or cricothyroid puncture (*see* Chapter 1). Anesthesia is induced using inhalational methods. Once fully anesthetized and all reflexes are abolished, intubation should be carried out. This process is very demanding and should only be carried out by those experienced in all aspects of pediatric airway care.

Once the airway is secure intravenous lines can be established, blood cultures and blood for other investigations taken, and treatment against *H. influenzae* B initiated according to local guidelines.

Should the child develop acute laryngospasm and airway obstruction, immediate cricothyroid puncture should be performed (*see* Chapter 1).

	Croup	**Epiglottitis**	**Inhaled foreign body**
Cause	Viral	Haemophilus inluenzae	Foreign body
Preceding illness	Coryzal	None	None
Onset	Slow	Rapid	Rapid
Associated signs	Harsh, barking cough	Quiet, drooling	Quiet, drooling
Systemic signs	Usually none	Toxic pyrexial	None

Figure 3.9
Clinical features associated with three common causes of stridor. These should be taken as a general guide only.

CROUP (LARYNGOTRACHEOBRONCHITIS)

It can be difficult at times to distinguish croup from epiglottitis. If there is any doubt about the diagnosis, the child should be treated as if epiglottitis is present.

Even if croup is diagnosed, increasing edema in the airways or superimposed bacterial infection may narrow the airway further. This in turn will lead to increasing respiratory distress and the child may in fact be intubated purely for relief of obstructive symptoms.

Occasionally, croup is complicated by superimposed bacterial infection typically leading to tracheitis. The child can be quite toxic and prolonged intubation and ventilation may be required together with regular tracheal suction.

Most children follow a benign, uncomplicated course and most can be managed safely at home. It is traditional to keep a child in a steam-filled room. There have, however, been a number of instances where the child has been scalded in these situations and great care should be taken if one is using boiling water to humidify the atmosphere. One way to avoid this is to run a hot bath and bring the child into the bathroom; this may be the safest option.

Increased respiratory distress is an indication to give the child nebulised adrenaline (epinephrine) with of without steroids. There is evidence to suggest that steroids given orally or by nebuliser may reduce edema enough to avoid ventilation.

This treatment option, however, requires that the child be kept for observation.

INHALED FOREIGN BODY

A history of choking, spluttering or transient distress in a child known to have had a foreign body, particularly a small object, in his or her mouth should be taken seriously.

Foreign bodies in the upper airway will usually be wedged in the larynx or just below at the level of the cricoid. These will almost invariably cause complete airway obstruction. In this situation a child will become comatose very quickly and should be treated according to the principles detailed in Chapter 2.

If the foreign body passes the vocal cords and the cricoid it will usually wedge somewhere around the carina or the right main bronchus (**Figure 3.11**). Often the foreign bodies are radiolucent and will not be visible on X-ray (**Figure 3.12 a**). A normal chest X-ray is found in 21% of children harboring an inhaled foreign body. A high index of suspicion is needed in this

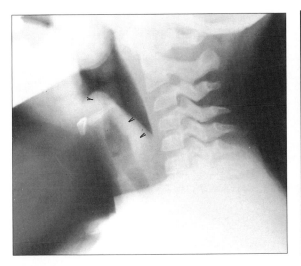

Figure 3.10
Lateral neck view indicating a swollen epiglottis (arrow) and aryepiglottic folds (arrowheads). The appearances are typical of epiglottitis—this condition is usually diagnosed clinically and with direct endoscopy. X-rays should only be performed in the ward or emergency room, in the erect position, and with full resuscitative measures available.

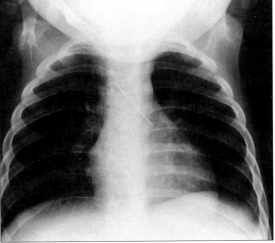

Figure 3.11
This 3-year-old child had aspirated a needle. The needle was shown to be lying in the left main bronchus. The appearances were confirmed with a lateral chest X-ray .

situation. It may be necessary to admit the child for observation and further imaging investigations such as inspiration/expiration films or chest fluoroscopy (**Figure 3.12 b**). Bronchoscopy will confirm the diagnosis and facilitate the foreign body.

It is difficult at times to determine whether the foreign body is in the airway or in the esophagus. Children who have swallowed ball bearings, large coins or other large bodies may have the object wedged in the esophagus. Symptoms may mimic partial airway obstruction at the level of the cricoid. The child will often drool and salivate excessively (**Figure 3.13**). A lateral X-ray is indicated. There is no urgency with regard to this situation as long as the child is maintaining an airway and breathing well.

PNEUMONIA

Pneumonia frequently follows upper respiratory tract infection. However, other causes, such as foreign body inhalation or pneumonitis, should be considered.

Typically, the child will present with coughing, often with a preceding history of respiratory tract infection. Abdominal pain is not infrequent and can be misleading. It is important to examine the chest in all children with abdominal pain and pyrexia.

The child is invariably toxic and it can be difficult to distinguish the signs of toxicity from the signs of pneumonia. Both of these include tachypnea, respiratory distress and grunting. Clinical examination in older children may reveal areas of consolidation characterized by dullness with or without crepitations. These signs can be difficult to obtain in smaller children.

If suspected, the child should have a chest X-ray which will reveal bronchopneumonia (patchy and diffuse infiltration) or lobar pneumonia (dense consolidation) (**Figure 3.14**). If in doubt the X-ray should be discussed, in selected cases, with the radiologist. The radiologist may recommend that lateral X-rays be taken as this may help localize the lobe involved.

Resistant lower lobe pneumonias without a history of preceding viral illness should lead one to consider the possibility of foreign body aspiration.

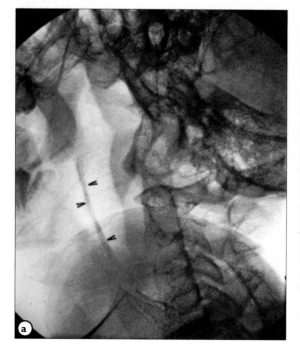

Figure 3.12 a

Foreign body in airway. This child choked on a plastic foreign body. Note the lodged linear foreign body lying in the oropharynx (arrowheads). This is clearly seen due to the contrast between air and the low density of the plastic.

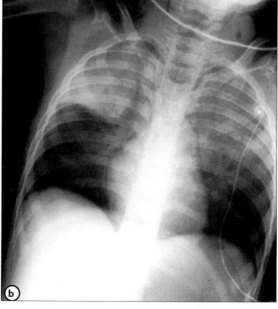

Figure 3.12 b Chest X-ray demonstrating complications of an aspirated foreign body. Both upper lobes show extensive consolidation with pulmonary edema. There is evidence of surgical emphysema of the neck. The child had choked on a sausage. Pulmonary edema associated with acute obstruction is well recognized and is thought to be due to the very high negative intrathoracic pressures on inspiration.

ORGANISMS

Staphylococcal infections have to be considered in children under 2 years of age along with *Streptococcus pneumoniae* and *H. influenzae*, which are common in all age groups. Gram-negative organisms are found much more frequently in infants than in older age groups.

Other causes of pneumonia need to be considered if the initial infection does not settle on conventional therapy. *Mycoplasma pneumoniae* can cause atypical infections unresponsive to penicillin. Outbreaks of mycoplasma come about cyclically so peaks and troughs occur. Most respond to erythromycin.

MANAGEMENT

The urgency and extent of treatment will depend on the toxicity of the child. As most of these children are systemically unwell, inpatient treatment should be actively considered, particularly for those under 1 year of age who may have Gram-negative organism or staphylococcal infection. Oxygen saturation should be monitored where possible and oxygen therapy provided if the saturation level falls below 95%. Intravenous access should be established and intravenous fluids given by this route if the child is dehydrated or not tolerating oral fluids. After blood cultures have been taken, intravenous antibiotics should be administered.

In children under 1 year of age, flucloxacillin and gentamicin should be prescribed to cover staphylococcus and coliforms. In older children penicillin or amoxycillin are the drugs of choice. Erythromycin may be needed if mycoplasma is implicated.

SUPPLEMENTARY INFORMATION

Additional information may be obtained from a full blood count. Blood cultures should be drawn for all toxic children. Mycoplasma and viral titres at presentation and after 10–14 days may help to confirm difficult cases. Blood for these titres can be drawn at initial presentation and stored for later analysis to avoid unnecessary expense. Only if clinical concern arises should further samples be sent for analysis.

DIFFERENTIAL DIAGNOSIS

The differential diagnosis should include other causes of respiratory distress and heart failure.

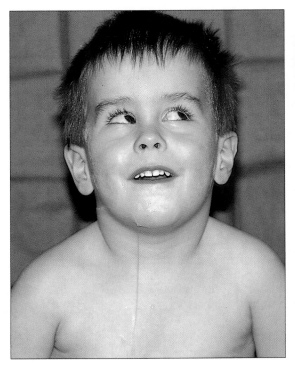

Figure 3.13
Foreign body in upper oesophagus. He is non-toxic and unable to swallow saliva. He has a foreign body in his oesophagus mimicking an airway obstruction.

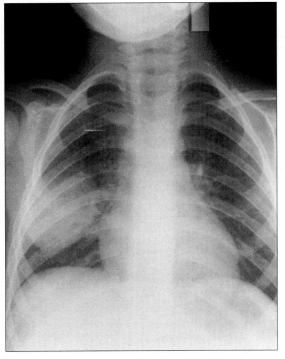

Figure 3.14
Posteroanterior chest X-ray in a child presenting with fever and cough. The X-ray demonstrates a 5 cm diameter coin lesion in the right lung. This is consistent with a pneumonia.

NEUROLOGIC EMERGENCIES

COMA

Comatose children attend the AED relatively infrequently compared with the adult population. It is important to have a coordinated approach to these children as the diagnoses are multitudinous.

All unconscious children are at risk from airway obstruction due to the tongue falling into the pharynx. The principles of treatment alluded to in the section on basic life support (*see* Chapters 1 and 2) should be established at a very early stage.

A useful mnemonic—AEIOUTIPS—may help with diagnosis (**Figure 3.15**).

APPROACH TO THE UNCONSCIOUS CHILD

The importance of stabilising the airway, breathing and circulation have already been covered (*see* Chapter 1). A rapid primary survey should be completed and a secondary survey performed to rule out the diagnoses detailed below. Any treatable lesion or condition should be dealt with urgently. This should be followed by a series of baseline investigations—these will obviously be directed by the result of the primary and secondary surveys.

Where trauma is suspected, it is important to treat the child as a trauma patient (*see* Trauma section: Chapter 4).

Baseline investigations should include:

- **Glucose:** this may help establish hypo/hyperglycemia. Stick testing by the bedside is a good screen, but formal samples should be sent for confirmation.
- **White cell count:** a raised white cell count may be associated with infection. Overwhelming sepsis may result in a low white cell count.
- **Urea and electrolytes:** this will often be normal but should be analyzed. A rise in potassium may be the first clue to renal failure.
- **Blood count:** one is looking for signs of decreased hematocrit (associated with hypovolemia) and low counts of platelets and hemoglobin (bleeding, leukemia, sepsis).
- **Clotting screen:** abnormalities may indicate liver derangement or a bleeding disorder which may in turn cause intracranial hemorrhage.
- **Blood culture:** to rule out sepsis (not of immediate value).
- **Blood:** for grouping and save serum
- **Spare sample:** to spin down and freeze for later, analysis of ammonia, insulin and enzyme deficiency associated with inborn errors of metabolism
- **Urine:** for culture, sensitivity and toxicology. A sample should be stored for later analysis for inborn errors of metabolism if required.
- **Skull X-ray:** if trauma is suspected.
- **Chest X-ray:** if infection or aspiration is suspected.
- **Blood gases:** metabolic derangement may show as acidosis. Also the adequacy of ventilation and perfusion can be assessed.

Once the child is safe, urgent admission to a high-dependency/intensive care unit should be arranged as soon as possible, via imaging, (for example CT scanning of the brain if indicated).

ALCOHOL

Alcohol intoxication is one of the most common reasons for people to be unconscious and this includes children and adolescents. Large numbers of children, particularly at party times such as Christmas and New Year, end up imbibing alcohol. Relatively small amounts can cause quite profound coma in these children. Not only are they prone to vomiting with resultant inhalation but they are also susceptible to hypoglycemia and hypothermia.

EPILEPSY

Children can have fits (or faints with subsequent epileptic attacks). Children who have had a fit may remain unconscious for some time. All the usual causes of epilepsy should be sought in these children. If the child is still fitting appropriate anticonvulsant therapy should be given (*see* **Figure 3.16**).

Predisposing causes of coma or altered consciousness in children
A   **A**lcohol
E   **E**pilepsy
I   **I**nsulin-related problems (hypo/hyperglycemia)
O   **O**verdose (deliberate)
U   **U**nusual (rare) metabolic problems
T   **T**rauma (and hypovolemia)
I   **I**ntracranial problems (e.g. meningitis/encephalitis/ intracranial hemorrhage)
P   **P**oisoning (accidental)
S   **S**epsis

Figure 3.15

INSULIN-RELATED PROBLEMS

Hypoglycemia is a relatively more common cause of coma than hyperglycemia. All children, whether they are known diabetics or not, who are unconscious should have their blood sugar level measured. Formal laboratory assessment will take some time to report but a bedside needle-stick test should be performed immediately. If the glucose level is low the child should be treated with glucose (*see* Metabolic Emergencies). If the child has normal or raised blood sugar, no harm will be done. On the other hand, if the blood sugar is high, treatment should not be started until a formal blood sugar is returned.

OVERDOSE (DELIBERATE)

This is an increasing problem in adolescent and teenage children. The child may deliberately take an overdose and subsequently try to hide the situation from relatives and other adults. The possibility that the child is also a secret substance abuser should be noted. It is important to liaise with the local toxicology department when dealing with unconscious children so that appropriate samples, either from gastric aspirate, blood or urine, can be sent for toxicologic analysis. While the pick up rate may be low, overdose is still an important diagnosis to exclude. Munchausen-by-proxy should also be considered in younger children.

UNUSUAL (RARE) METABOLIC CAUSES

Young children with Reyes syndrome may present with a raised ammonia level, hypoglycemia and deepening level of unconsciousness associated with liver failure.

Infants with a hitherto undiagnosed inborn error of metabolism may only present as an unconscious child after a challenge such as infection. These inborn errors can effect any of the pathways of glucose, fat and protein metabolism. In these children it is important that blood and urine be sent for metabolite screening. Subsequent tests may need to be conducted and these samples may be the only confirmatory specimens available. This should not delay appropriate treatment and resuscitation.

TRAUMA AND HYPOVOLEMIA

Trauma may result in either head injury, occult internal bleeding or both. Any of these situations can result in the child having an altered level of consciousness. Evidence of head injury should be sought, namely obvious bruising and signs of base-of-skull fracture.

Signs of hypovolemia manifest as poor peripheral circulation, cold peripheries etc. (*see* Chapter 1). Similarly, hypovolemia may also be attributed to cardiogenic, anaphylactic or septic causes.

INTRACRANIAL PROBLEMS

The possibility of encephalitis, meningitis and intracranial hematoma should all be considered.

The possibility of non-accidental injury in a small child should not be ignored. Retinal hemorrhages may be associated with the 'shaken baby syndrome' (*see* section on Non-Accidental injury).

A CT scan may be helpful in these situations demonstrating intracranial haemorrhage. Magnetic resonance imaging is more accurate in dating bleeding and in the detection of parenchymal damge.

POISONING (ACCIDENTAL)

Children, particularly young children, often find pills, potions and household products that may render them unconscious. As with deliberate overdose, this may not be appreciated early in the diagnosis. A high index of suspicion is necessary and parents should be asked to check the possibility of the child having had access to noxious substances. The possibility of carbon monoxide poisoning should also be considered—this may be indicated by the child having a cherry-red appearance and abnormally high pulse oximeter readings.

SEPSIS

This will include meningitis and septic shock. The child may be pyrexial and have a bounding pulse but still exhibit evidence of relative hypovolemia. A petechial rash may be present.

FITS AND SEIZURES

Many different types of seizure activity present at the AED. The most common, however, is the generalized grand mal seizure. Most are either idiopathic or fever-related. Occasionally, trauma is a cause. No matter what the cause, the principles of treatment are the same:

- Ensuring airway, breathing and circulation are secure.
- Administration of appropriate anticonvulsant therapy.
- Appropriate investigations.
- Appropriate disposal.

IDIOPATHIC GRAND MAL SEIZURES

These can occur in a child *de novo* or can occur in a child already diagnosed as having epilepsy. In the former situation, treatment should be reasonably straight forward and follow the accompanying scheme (**Figure 3.16**). The only addition to children who have established epilepsy is to ensure that anticonvulsant blood levels are measured. Many of these children may have inadequate anticonvulsant levels for various reasons and this needs to be considered as a matter of urgency. It is important to make sure that there is no new underlying cause such as electrolyte imbalance or hypoglycemia. The management of grand mal seizures is summarized in **Figure 3.16**.

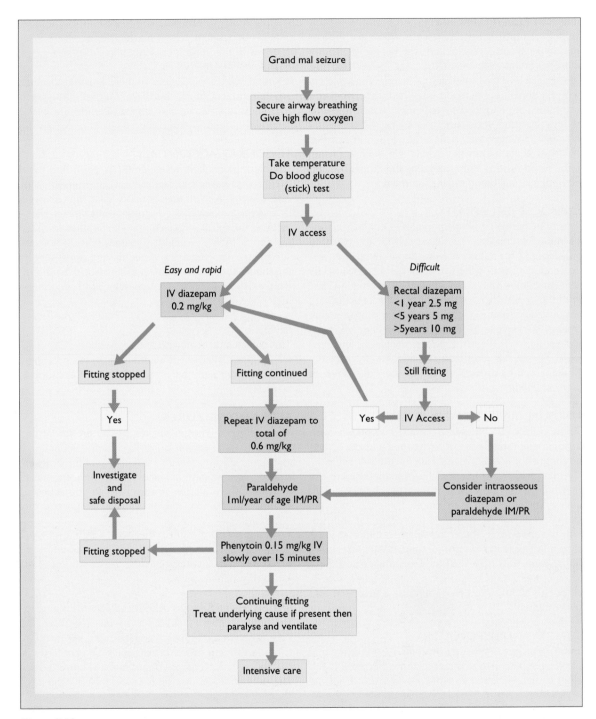

Figure 3.16
Algorithm for treatment of Grand Mal Seizure.

FEBRILE CONVULSION

This is the most common cause of seizure in the under 5s age group. The etiology is unknown. It is a very worrying and distressing situation for parents to see a child fitting. In panic, it is not unusual for parents to put a fitting child in the back of a car and drive across the city to an AED. A major aim of first aid programs should be to try and dissuade parents from this action—they should be instructed in the basic care of fitting children and told to call an ambulance.

The principles of treatment follow that for any grand mal seizure. Only if the child is still fitting on arrival should any treatment be offered apart from antipyretic measures.

Children who have febrile convulsions associated with prolonged seizures, i.e. greater than 5 minutes, should be taken more seriously than those with brief febrile seizures. Most will have an obvious focus for infection although rare causes include appendicitis, osteomyelitis and other hidden sepsis. A search should be made for the focus of infection. Local policies will decide whether this should include a lumbar puncture. Very few children will have meningitis.

All first febrile seizures should be admitted for a short period of observation if only for the parents' peace of mind.

The child should be observed for evidence that the pyrexia is settling and that there is no sign of significant infection as detailed above. The child can then be discharged, with advice to the parents on how to relieve pyrexia and to deal with a febrile fit should it happen again.

Only if the seizures are repeated or recurrent should anticonvulsant therapy be considered.

ISOLATED NERVE PALSIES

The external eye muscles are supplied by cranial nerves, numbers III, IV, and VI.

Most cases of ocular muscle palsy are congenital but occasionally can present *de novo*. The differential diagnosis will include:
- Head trauma.
- Tumor.
- Raised intracranial pressure, for example hydrocephalus, cerebral edema.
- Meningitis.
- Cavernous sinus thrombosis.

All children with a spontaneous onset of external ocular muscle palsy must be referred as a matter of urgency to either a neurologist or neurosurgeon, according to local practice. The child will almost certainly require further investigation which will include either CT scanning or MRI.

SEVENTH NERVE PALSY

Seventh nerve palsy or Bell's palsy is relatively common in childhood (**Figure 3.17**). Usually no predisposing cause is found, though one should be sought. Predisposing causes will include:
- Head trauma.
- Middle ear infection.
- Ramsay Hunt syndrome.

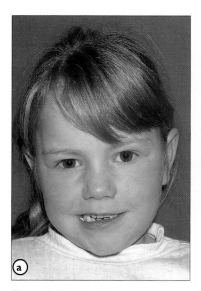 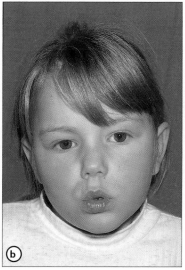 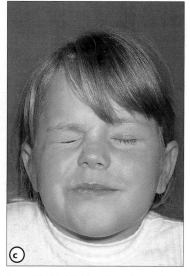

Figure 3.17 a, b and c
This young girl has a left-sided facial weakness due to a seventh nerve palsy (Bell's palsy). No abnormality is noted until she tries to smile (a) or whistle (b), then a left-sided facial weakness is noted. (c) When she closes her eyes the left eye does not close as tightly as the right.

Ramsay Hunt syndrome is an inflammation of the facial nerves secondary to herpes infection. Classically, there will be facial paralysis, with vesicles along the line of the seventh nerve in the pinna or the external auditory meatus. Should Ramsay Hunt syndrome be present immediate referral to an ENT specialist should be made.

Otherwise treatment should be expectant. There is no proven evidence that steroids will work, particularly if given after 48 hours. Most cases of seventh-nerve palsy resolve spontaneously after a period of 3–4 weeks. Follow-up is required to ensure resolution is complete; this will depend on local facilities and interests.

MENINGITIS

Meningitis is one of the most feared infections of our time. While it is exceedingly rare, it causes significant morbidity and mortality. Meningitis can be classified as follows:

- Bacterial.
- Viral.
- Atypical.

BACTERIAL MENINGITIS

Common organisms responsible for meningitis include *Neisseria meningitidis*, *S. pneumoniae* and *H. influenzae*. Since immunization has been instituted, *H. influenzae* infection is becoming less prevalent. In the neonatal period, coliform organisms must be added to this list of pathogens.

Symptoms and signs of bacterial meningitis are legion and seldom do the classic symptoms of headache, photophobia and neck stiffness present. This is particularly true in the neonatal period where such diffuse symptoms as apneic attacks, 'off-feeds' and vomiting can be significant presenting complaints.

Physical examination in younger children can be equally disappointing. The presence or absence of a bulging fontanelle is neither reassuringly positive nor negative. A strong index of suspicion, therefore, is needed before the diagnosis of meningitis can be confidently excluded. If there is any doubt at all about the possibility of meningitis being present, a lumbar puncture is the only certain way of excluding the diagnosis.

In children who are comatose or who have had a seizure, lumbar puncture should be avoided and empiric treatment initiated, pending cranial imaging.

Children who have *N. meningitidis* meningitis do not invariably have meningococcal septicemia. In these situations a typical purpuric rash may well be absent.

VIRAL MENINGITIS

Viral meningitis is as perplexing as a bacterial diagnosis. Again, the only definite method of diagnosis is analysis of CSF following lumbar puncture.

ATYPICAL MENINGITIS

Included among this category are tuberculous meningitis and listeria meningitis. These are exceedingly rare and beyond the scope of this text to discuss further.

MANAGEMENT OF MENINGITIS

Once meningitis is suspected, a lumbar puncture should be performed as soon as possible (**Figure 3.18**). A lumbar puncture should not be performed in children who have an altered level of consciousness, a raised intracranial pressure, or have fitted. In these situations empiric treatment should be started and appropriate measures to alleviate intracranial pressure commenced.

Lumbar puncture should be performed using an aseptic technique. If an atraumatic tap is made, a brief

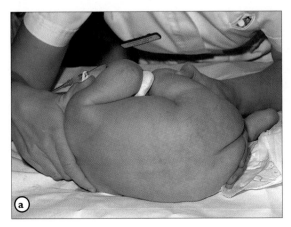

Figure 3.18 a
A child in the correct position for a lumbar puncture. A nurse pulls the child into full flexion and holds the child securely in place in the left lateral position.

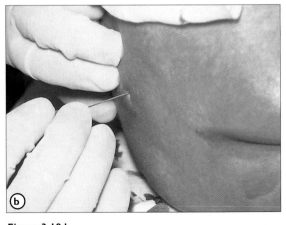

Figure 3.18 b
A lumbar puncture needle is inserted perpendicular to the spine and pushed slowly forwards until a give is felt. The trochar is then removed and the cerebrospinal fluid collected.

examination of the fluid with the naked eye can be helpful. Turbid fluid may suggest infection, but infected fluid is not always turbid.

Empiric treatment should be commenced against all the organisms mentioned above. Penicillin combined with a third generation cephalosporin are an appropriate combination of antibiotics, although local policies should be followed.

H. influenzae infection is associated with deafness. The incidence of postmeningitis hearing problems can be significantly reduced if steroids are initiated early in the course of the infection. Streptococcal and meningococcal meningitis are associated much less frequently with hearing damage and it is debatable whether steroids are of benefit in these situations.

With the introduction of *H. influenzae* vaccination, the rate of infection from this organism has fallen and therefore also the need for steroids.

CARDIAC DISEASE

Two broad categories of cardiac problems present to the AED:
- Heart failure.
- Cardiac dysrhythmia.

Often these conditions will coexist.

HEART FAILURE
This usually presents in infancy, mainly as a result of underlying congenital heart disease. In older children there may be an underlying condition, typically a myocarditis or cardiomyopathy (**Figure 3.19**), although congenital lesions also occur. Extra cardiac causes should be sought, for example, renal failure (**Figure 3.20**).

Clinical features in young children can be varied. The similarities between chest infection and heart failure make a diagnosis difficult to achieve at times (**Figure 3.21**).

PRINCIPLES OF TREATMENT
Treatment is directed at correcting any underlying cause and normalising the circulation as soon as possible.

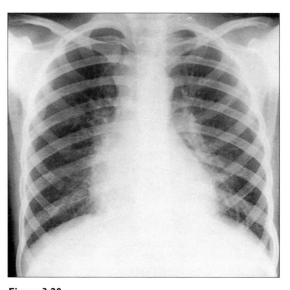

Figure 3.20
Chest X-ray in a child with acute glomerulonephritis. The heart is enlarged. The lung fields show a reticular pattern with septal lines at the bases and a small left pleural effusion. Appearances are consistent with interstitial pulmonary edema.

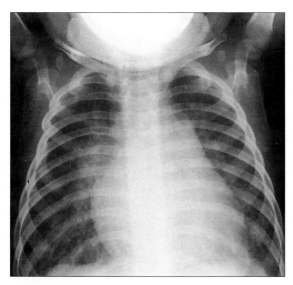

Figure 3.19
Posteroanterior chest X-ray of a child with rapid onset of pulmonary edema, secondary to cardiomyopathy. Note the enlarged heart, and reticular nodular pattern in the lung fields indicative of interstitial pulmonary edema.

Symptoms and signs of heart failure	
Symptoms	Signs
Exhaustion–particularly when feeding	Tachycardia
Rapid breathing	Gallop rhythym
Cold peripheries	Hepatomegaly
Excess weight gain	Edema–particularly in dependent areas
Cyanosis	

Figure 3.21

Careful attention should be paid to the airway, breathing and circulation. The mainstay of treatment is oxygenation and diuretic therapy; fluid restriction (two-thirds of the daily requirement) may help.

If there is any evidence of hypoxia the child should be treated with oxygen. Keeping the child semi-erect may help reduce symptoms. Intravenous access should be established early.

Early investigations will include:
- 12-lead electrocardiography (ECG).
- Chest X-ray.
- Blood gases.
- Urea and electrolytes.
- Blood culture.
- Hemoglobin.

The role of digoxin is unclear. If used, digitalization should be achieved slowly over 24–48 hours orally. The intravenous route should be used if oral therapy is not possible.

While it is important to start treatment early, this should be done in full consultation with a cardiologist.

Children who are in full cardiogenic shock will usually require artificial ventilation to maintain oxygenation. Inotropic support with dopamine or dobutamine will also be required. This should be discussed with the receiving cardiologist and pediatric intensivist.

CARDIAC DYSRHYTHMIAS

Two common dysrhythmias occur in childhood:
- Tachycardia.
- Bradycardia.

These are in addition to the collapse rhythms of asystole, ventricular fibrillation and electromechanical dissociation which have been discussed under cardiac arrest (*see* Chapter 2).

TACHYCARDIA

Tachycardia is common in children in an AED setting. Usually this is an appropriate 'fight or flight' response. Tachycardia has many causes:
- Pyrexia/infection.
- Fear.
- Pain.
- Hypoxia.
- Hypovolemia.
- Heart failure.
- Cardiac conduction defects.
- Poisoning.

SUPRAVENTRICULAR TACHYCARDIA (SVT)
(Figure 3.22)

This is relatively common in infancy. It may be associated with an anomalous pre-excitation pathway as in the Wolfe–Parkinson–White syndrome. Once diagnosed, a brief assessment of the state of the child should be made.

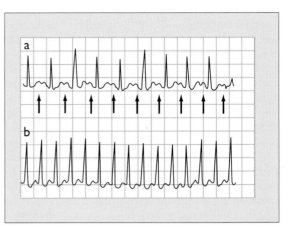

Figure 3.22
a. Sinus tachycardia rate. Note 'P-waves' before each 'QRS' compiler.
b. Supraventrical tachycardia rate. Note the faster rate than A and 'P-waves' are absent.

Either the child will be:
- In mild or minimal distress.
- In moderate distress.
- In severe distress.

Treatment will vary according to the underlying state of the child.

Mild or minimal distress

The older child will often be awake and talking. There may be some chest discomfort. Infants seldom present this way. Typically, there will be a period of increasing malaise and poor feeding, often diagnosed as viral illness.

Treatment

One can try to abort the SVT with vagal stimulation maneuvers. These are usually ineffective in the older child who may well have tried them at home. Immersing the infant's head in cold water or applying an ice pack to the face can be effective though these latter maneuvers need a lot of explanation to the parents! Adenosine, 100 µg/kg rising to 250 µg/kg in 50 µg/kg boluses, can also be effective. In this situation a dose of 200 µg/kg makes the child feel uncomfortable with significant gastric side-effects. In such situations disopyramide 2–3 mg/kg given slowly over 10 minutes and with ECG control may be effective.

MODERATE DISTRESS

Here the child will display signs such as mild hypotension and there may be peripheral shut down (*see* Chapter 1). Blood pressure will usually be normal. In these situations Adenosine may again be of benefit, but with the same problems already described.

SEVERE DISTRESS

In this situation the child exhibits signs of profound shock and hypotension. The child should be resuscitated ensuring attention to the airway, breathing and circulation (*see* Chapter 1). The child should be oxygenated effectively and intravenous access secured rapidly.

One should consider synchronized direct current (DC) cardioversion under sedation as a matter of urgency. While waiting for sedation to be achieved, it may be possible to abort the attack with adenosine in the doses stated above. However, if the child is profoundly shocked and deteriorating rapidly, synchronized DC cardioversion should take place without delay.

ADENOSINE

Adenosine should be given as a very rapid IV injection followed immediately by a 'push' of normal saline. One reason for adenosine to fail is injecting too slowly.

WIDE COMPLEX TACHYCARDIA (Figure 2.10)

Wide complex tachycardia is occasionally a cause for confusion. The differential diagnosis is either that of supraventricular tachycardia with aberrant conduction or ventricular tachycardia. As a principle, ventricular arrhythmias are rare in pediatric practice.

Ventricular tachycardia will either present in a child who is stable or unstable, as defined by level of consciousness, respiratory function and particularly the state of the circulation (*see* Chapter 1).

If the child has collapsed the rhythm should be treated as for ventricular fibrillation (*see* Chapter 2). If the child is stable it is worth trying Adenosine as directed above. If the child responds, the rhythm is probably supraventricular with aberrant conduction. Failure to respond will lead to a diagnosis of ventricular tachycardia, which may be treated with lignocaine (lidocaine) 1 mg/kg followed by an infusion of 0.2 mg/kg/minute. Synchronized DC cardioversion may also be tried, particularly if signs of decompensation occur.

BRADYCARDIA (Figure 3.23)

A child with sinus bradycardia usually has an underlying cause. This will most often be due to hypoxia and/or hypovolemia, as discussed previously. These should be sought and if present actively treated as previously discussed in Chapter 1.

One also has to consider raised intracranial pressure and the possibility of drug ingestion.

In cases of drug ingestion no treatment should be considered unless the child is symptomatic. In other situations, the underlying cause should be sought and treated aggressively.

Bradycardia secondary to underlying cardiac abnormalities may respond to either epinephrine or atropine in appropriate doses. Pacing, either internal or external, may also be considered.

RENAL DISORDERS

Renal disorders are very common in childhood and four types can be recognised:
- Acute renal failure.
- Glomerulitis.
- Hematuria.
- Urinary tract infection.

ACUTE RENAL FAILURE

Acute renal failure is characterized by a decrease in urinary output and rising urea and creatinine levels. A urine output of 1 ml/kg/hour is considered adequate for most children and anything below this for a prolonged period of time should be classified as a decreased urine output.

This scenario rarely presents to the AED. It takes time to empty the bladder initially. Even if $^1/_2$-hourly urine volumes are estimated subsequently it will take 1–2 hours to detect a diminished output compatible with renal failure.

More especially, renal failure should be suspected in children presenting with acute heart failure (**Figure 3.20**), post-seizure or comatose. In these children, underlying disease predisposing to renal failure may be found by taking a careful history and making an examination following the initial primary and resuscitation phases (*see* Chapter 1) (**Figure 3.24**).

The net result of the decreased urine outflow is twofold:
- Pulmonary edema and fluid overload from the inability to excrete fluid.
- Electrolyte imbalance leading to severe life-threatening hyperkalemia.

Associated with these may be hypertension and seizures (due to metabolic derangement or hypertensive encephalopathy).

While the role of the AED should not be ignored, a full discussion on the management of renal failure is beyond the scope of this text.

Initially a brief history can be obtained and some clue as to the predisposing cause of the renal failure can be established.

Prerenal failure can be suspected if there is a history of blood loss, vomiting and/or diarrhea or cardiac failure.

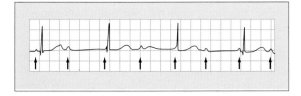

Figure 3.23

Bradycardia Palpable pulse= 47 beats/min. Ventricular rate on ECG = 47 complexes/min. P waves (arrows) do not relate to ventricular activation (QRS complexes) and occur at a regular rate of 93/min.

Causes of renal failure		
Prerenal	Renal	Post-renal
Diarrhea	Glomerulonephritis	Urethral valves
Vomiting	Antibiotic toxicity	Trauma
Cardiac failure	Heavy metal poisoning	Tumor
Hemorrhage	Rhabdomyolysis	Obstruction at PUJ and VUJ
Burns	Hemolytic uremic syndrome	

Figure 3.24

Renal causes of renal failure should be suspected if there is a history of streptococcal tonsillitis (leading to poststreptococcal nephritis), hematuria, systemic disease such as Henoch–Schoenlein purpura, recent antibiotic administration (e.g. aminoglycoside) or other unusual events. Preceding diarrhea, especially containing blood, may be a harbinger of Hemolytic Uremic Syndrome.

Postrenal renal failure should be suspected in a child with known reflux or renal obstruction, trauma or other disorders of the postrenal tract.

Hypoxia and hypovolemia should be treated as detailed previously (*see* Chapter 1). An urgent urea, electrolytes, creatinine and blood gas estimation should be obtained. A 12-lead ECG may give early clues to the presence of hyperkalemia (**Figure 3.25**).

If acidosis is severe, bicarbonate should be administered but it is important to avoid fluid and sodium overload in this situation. Severe hyperkalemia should be treated with insulin and dextrose. Calcium gluconate given intravenously may also help counter the toxic effects of a raised potassium level. Calcium resonium ions, 0.5 g/kg, will help increase potassium elimination. The child should be admitted to a high-dependency area as soon as possible.

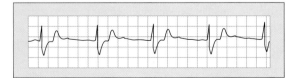

Figure 3.25
Hyperkalaemia. Note that there are no P-Waves. Broad QRS complexes (b). Tall peaked T waves. This child had a potassium of 7.8 and was suffering from renal failure 2° to Haemolytic uremic syndrome.

There are reports of salbutamol being effective in reducing serum potassium levels. The standard treatment of insulin and dextrose has stood the test of time. There is some concern over administering a potentially cardiotoxic drug (salbutamol) to a myocardium already at risk of arrhythmia from raised plasma potassium levels.

GLOMERULONEPHRITIS

Glomerulonephritis is an immune disorder of the kidneys typically following previous infection. Streptococci, other bacteria and viruses are implicated.

Typically, the child will present with slight puffiness around the eyes, often noticed by members of the family. Vague abdominal symptoms may be present. Urine testing will show hematuria with proteinuria. Blood pressure may be raised and laboratory investigations will reveal raised plasma urea and plasma creatinine levels. Once diagnosed, the child should be referred for an urgent pediatric opinion when further investigation and treatment can be considered.

Significant renal impairment is rare in the early stages of glomerulonephritis but occasionally children present with renal failure which should be dealt with as above.

MACROSCOPIC HEMATURIA

The presence of frank or altered blood in the urine (hematuria) is a symptom that causes great alarm in the child and the parents. Causes include:
- Trauma.
- Infection.
- Glomerulonephritis.
- Bleeding disorder.
- Tumor, for example Wilms tumor.

Macroscopic hematuria following trauma should lead one to consider significant renal tract damage (*see* Abdominal Trauma: Chapter 4). After the 'ABC' of resuscitation has been carried out, and the child is stable, further investigation of the renal tract can be organized by the pediatric radiologist. This will include ultrasound with doppler, intravenous urography and CT.

Atraumatic causes of hematuria should be taken seriously. Firstly, the hematuria should be confirmed by both dipstick testing (**Figure 3.26**) and by microscopic examination of the urine. If confirmed, the child should be referred to the pediatric team for further urgent investigation. Baseline parameters, such as blood pressure, should be documented.

Simple investigations to be carried out in the AED include a full blood count, blood culture, coagulation screen, and group and save serum. This is particularly important in cases of bleeding diathesis, when further treatment may be needed urgently, either to increase coagulation or to replace blood loss.

Streptococcal and viral causes of nephritis may be associated with altered serology. Consequently, serum should also be sent for further analysis.

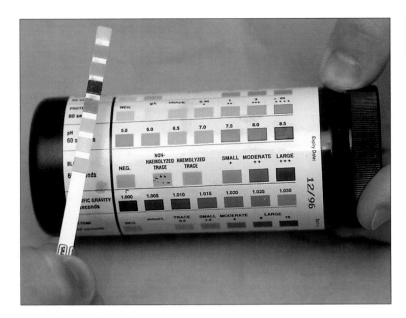

Figure 3.26
Dipstick testing of urine will reveal hematuria, proteinuria and glycosuria.

MICROSCOPIC HEMATURIA

Microscopic hematuria has many causes, many of which are benign. It can follow exercise or a febrile illness of extrarenal etiology. More commonly, the urine will be contaminated with blood from the genital area. This can occur in menstruating girls or if there has been minor urethral trauma.

Hematuria associated with proteinuria should be taken more seriously. While infection is more likely to be the cause, glomerulonephritis may also be present.

URINARY TRACT INFECTION

Urinary tract infections are a common cause of pyrexia, abdominal pain and vomiting in children. Young children and infants will seldom complain of dysuria. **As such, all pyrexial infants should have their urine tested with a dipstick, particularly if no obvious cause is found on general examination.**

If urinary tract infection is suspected a urine sample should be obtained under sterile conditions (suprapubic tap if necessary) and divided into two samples. The first should be tested using a multitest dipstick and the second sent for urgent microscopy and culture. A positive dipstick test, i.e. blood and protein, indicates infection, particularly if other causes (*see* above) are excluded. Newer dipsticks are available which also test for leucocytes and nitrates. These are reliable indicators of infection.

The second sample should be kept sterile and sent to the laboratory for direct microscopy (the urgency of which will be determined from the condition of the child) and culture. Microscopy may show sufficient evidence for empiric treatment to be initiated pending full culture and sensitivity results. These results take a day or two to return

so it is sensible to start empiric treatment with antibiotics according to local sensitivity patterns. The child should be reviewed after a few days when the results of the culture and, hopefully, sensitivity analysis are available.

At this stage it will be clear if there is a urinary tract infection present and appropriate changes in treatment can be advised. All children with proven urinary tract infection should be referred for further investigation of the urinary tract (**Figure 3.27**).

The imaging modalities used in the investigation of the urinary tract are tailored to the age of the child. Ultrasound is a good baseline examination in all to exclude congenital abnormalities for example hydronephrosis, and complicated duplex kidneys. A Micturating Cystourethrogram (MCU) is necessary in the under 2 year old to detect and classify reflux and rule out urethral obstruction.

Radioisotope scans with T_c^{99m} MAG 3 provide time activity curves of passage of isotope through the kidneys

Under 1 year	US, MCU and DMSA scan
2–5 years	US, MAG3 isotope with voiding and DSMA
5 years +	US ± DMSA isotope scan

Figure 3.27
Investigation of first urinary tract infection by age of child.

and excretion. Delayed excretion and obstruction can be functionally evaluated. A MAG 3 voiding study can follow once the bladder is full of isotope. Reflux into the kidneys is manifest by peaks of activity in the renal areas. This technique is of value only in the older child who is toilet trained. T_c^{99m} DMSA injected IV is fixed to the tubular cells and can be used to estimate differential renal tissue function. It is a sensitive technique to detect renal scarring.

DIABETIC PROBLEMS

Children with diabetes are prone to either **hypoglycemia** or **ketoacidosis**. Hypoglycemia itself can be associated with other conditions:
- Excess insulin.
- Inborn error of metabolism.
- Reye's syndrome.
- Liver disease.
- Sepsis.
- Alcohol intoxication.

HYPOGLYCEMIA
Small children, particularly when ill or stressed, are more prone to hypoglycemia than older children due to their inadequate reserves of glycogen. For this reason they rapidly get exhausted and tired.

Hypoglycemia should be suspected in all unconscious children. If the blood sugar on a dipstick test reading is less than 2 mmol/litre then treatment should be started. **If at all possible blood should be taken for blood glucose analysis. Additional samples should be stored, especially in infants in whom inborn errors of metabolism are suspected**. These early untreated samples may be the only ones from which a diagnosis can be made (*see* Coma: Chapter 3).

HYPOGLYCEMIA IN DIABETIC CHILDREN
The treatment offered will be dependent on the clinical condition of the child. If the child is conscious and able to cooperate, a drink or tablet containing glucose may be all that is required. If the child is unconscious, or has insufficient gag reflexes present to protect the airway, parenteral therapy is indicated. **If intravenous access is readily established blood should be taken for dipstick analysis and also sent to the laboratory for formal investigation**. Dextrose 250 mg/kg (2.5 ml/kg 10% dextrose or 1 ml/kg 25% dextrose) should be given intravenously as a bolus over 5–10 minutes followed by a dextrose infusion. The response to this should be monitored.

If intravenous access is not readily established a bolus of glucagon should be administered intramuscularly; a dose of 1 mg can be used and repeated if there is no response after 20 minutes. Caution should be exercised when using glucagon as it relies on mobilizing glucose from store. If there is insufficient glucose in store it will not work as effectively.

An underlying cause for hypoglycemia should be sought and treated appropriately. Occasionally there will be a problem with insulin dosage. The possibility of either attempted suicide or Munchausen-by-proxy, while both rare, should always be considered.

KETOACIDOSIS
This is often the first presentation of a child with diabetes mellitus. Leading up to admission the child will complain of increasing thirst, polyuria and possibly malaise. Abdominal pain is also a feature. There may also be a period of weight loss. Children with poorly controlled diabetes are more prone to ketocidosis.

PATHOPHYSIOLOGY
A brief description of the pathophysiology of ketoacidosis is necessary to understand the main points of treatment. Basically, there is an inability of the body to metabolize glucose due to lack of insulin. This results in a build up of glucose in the blood which is eventually excreted into the urine. The presence of low molecular weight substances, such as glucose in the urine, act as osmotic stimulants and large amounts of fluid are drawn into the urinary system and the bladder thus causing polyuria. The net result is a relative dehydration of initially the intravascular space followed by the interstitial space and finally the intracellular space. The body recognizes itself as being dehydrated thus giving rise to thirst and polydipsia.

Because the body cannot use glucose as its substrate it turns to fat and protein metabolism. This leads to ketometabolism being switched on. Ketones are acidic in nature and lead to the metabolic acidosis which in turn aggravates the underlying metabolic disturbance. Insulin is required to maintain intracellular potassium. Lack of insulin will also increase potassium levels (**Figure 3.28**).

In known diabetics ketoacidosis can be precipitated by an increase in metabolic demand, such as that caused by infection or trauma, where insulin levels may not be adequate to meet the competing challenge of epinephrine (adrenaline) and other catabolic hormones. It should be possible to anticipate problems in these situations.

Biochemical findings in diabetic ketoacidosis
1. Hyperglycemia
2. Hyperkalemia
3. Ketones in the blood and breath
4. Rising hydrogen ion concentration in the blood
5. Increase in ketone and glucose in the urine

Figure 3.28

Principles for the treatment of diabetic ketoacidosis include:

- Restoration of circulatory volume.
- Restoration of glucose metabolism.
- Correction of electrolyte and other metabolic aberrations.
- Treatment of underlying cause.

Restoration of circulatory volume

Patients with diabetic ketoacidosis are usually quite severely volume depleted. There is good evidence that over-rapid infusion of fluid can result in intractable cerebral edema. It is important, therefore, to achieve a balance between the restoration of circulatory volume and an avoidance of a persistent hypovolemic state.

The child should be assessed for fluid loss and dehydration and treated according to **Figure 3.29**.

Initial fluid therapy in ketoacidosis		
Clinical signs	Fluid volume	Time
Shocked or greater than 10% dehydrated	Plasma 20 mls/kg	30–45 mins
5–10% dehydrated	Normal saline	30–45 mins

Figure 3.29

The next aim is to correct the dehydration over a 24 hour period. It is important to calculate the maintenance requirements for a normal child plus the fluid deficit. This total should then be divided by 24 which will give the hourly infusion rate. This should be given as normal saline until the blood sugar is below 13 mmol/l. Thereafter fluids should be given as 0.45% saline/5% dextrose.

Restoration of glucose metabolism

The mainstay of glucose metabolism is insulin. A slow intravenous infusion of insulin at a rate of 0.05 U/kg/hour should be initiated.

Once the infusion has been started blood sugar levels should be measured hourly.

Electrolytes

Potassium should be monitored carefully. Potassium should be added to the infusion at a rate of 20 mmol/500 ml once the child has been seen to pass urine.

The acidosis will respond to insulin and fluid therapy in the vast majority of cases. There is no place for bicarbonate therapy unless the child is very acidotic (e.g. pH<7.0).

Investigation

It is important to send for the following investigations as soon as possible:

- . Full blood count.
- Urea and electrolytes.
- Blood glucose.
- Blood osmolarity.
- Blood cultures.
- Blood gas analysis.

Sending for these should not delay resuscitation of the child and instigation of treatment.

Treatment of any underlying or precipitating cause

A cause for the ketoacidosis should be sought. This may involve a search for infection; throat swabs, urine culture, blood culture and swabs from any obvious septic lesion should be sent for analysis as necessary. The need for a chest X-ray should be based on clinical grounds as opposed to routine practice. A lumbar puncture will usually not be indicated in the first instance.

Further management

Treatment in the AED should not take more than 45–60 minutes. The child should be transferred as soon as possible to a high-dependency unit where further progress can be monitored.

ANAPHYLAXIS/ALLERGIC REACTIONS

The progression of acute allergic reactions into acute anaphylaxis is one of the problem areas of pediatric practice. Certainly, large numbers of children will present annually with various allergic manifestations, but only a few of these will proceed to develop full-blown anaphylaxis. It is important to predict those at risk.

ALLERGIC REACTIONS

Allergic reactions present in a variety of ways. These include:

- Urticaria.
- Rhinitis/conjunctivitis.
- Bronchospasm.
- Any combination of the above.

Usually all that is required is symptomatic treatment and withdrawal of the antigen wherever possible.
Unfortunately, it is not always possible to identify the antigen.

Simple urticaria should be treated with oral antihistamine. Occasionally, if the child is very severely distressed, parenteral therapy can be given (**Figure 3.30**). Treatment is continued for 2–3 days with subsequent follow-up by the child's doctor. Severe cases require treatment with corticosteroids, for example prednisolone 2 mg/kg for 3 days.

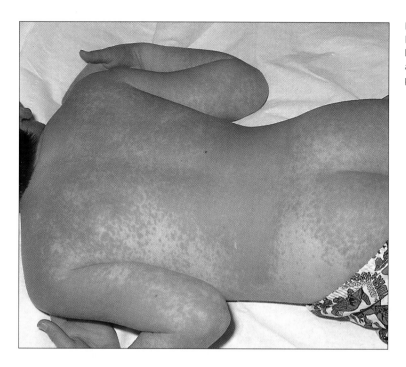

Figure 3.30
Marked urticaria over the trunk and upper legs. The mother had washed underwear in a new detergent to which the child is probably allergic.

Rhinitis and conjunctivitis can be more problematic. Nasal sprays containing corticosteroid used according to the manufacturer's directions may help in the treatment of rhinitis.

Conjunctivitis may be infective in nature and for that reason corticosteroids should not be used unless infection is excluded. Oral antihistamine may be effective. Should the problem not resolve within 24 hours, referral to an ophthalmologist may be required.

Bronchospasm is more serious and should be treated like any other asthma attack. Nebulized β_2-agonists and steroids are given as for asthma (*see* earlier).

ANGIONEUROTIC EDEMA

Angioneurotic edema is a more significant allergic reaction than the milder forms discussed above. Mild forms manifest simply as puffy eyes with slightly blotchy skin (**Figure 3.31**). This may progress rapidly to full-blown intra-oral and laryngeal edema.

Mild cases of puffy eyes, blotchy skin and **no** airway problems are treated with oral antihistamine and oral steroids. Treatment should continue for 3 days with each drug. The urine should be checked for protein to ensure a nephrotic syndrome or some other renal problem is not missed.

Fully developed angioneurotic edema with significant airway edema should be treated as follows: after securing the airway, drug therapy is commenced. This will include:

1. Epinephrine (adrenaline) 1:1000 per 0.1 mg/kg intramuscularly/intravenously.
2. Hydrocortisone 4 mg/kg intravenously.

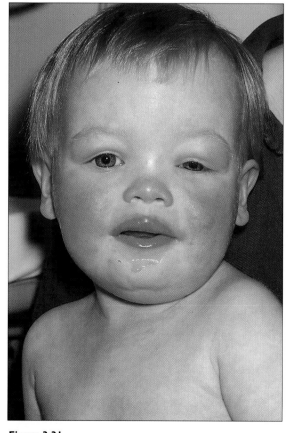

Figure 3.31
This child has puffy eyes and lips, and some irritation to her cheeks. She was playing with a pet dog and the swelling began shortly after.

Intravenous access should be secured as soon as possible. Steroid administration can be delayed until this has been achieved. There is no indication to wait for epinephrine to be administered and this should be given immediately.

The child should be transferred to a high-dependency unit as a matter of urgency.

ANAPHYLACTIC SHOCK

This is a systemic manifestation to an antigen, usually of unknown etiology. Any of the above characteristics of urticaria, bronchospasm, or angioneurotic edema may be present, but in association there is profound systemic collapse.

TREATMENT

The airway should be secured and intravenous access obtained as a matter of urgency. Epinephrine and hydrocortisone should be given as above. There will also be a need for fluid replacement, often on a massive scale. The child should be transferred to a high-dependency unit as soon as possible.

GASTROENTERITIS

Gastric upset, either isolated diarrhea or vomiting or a combination, is quite common in childhood. It is particularly prevalent in developing countries.

As with many other conditions, treatment will depend on the actual condition of the child and the parents ability to cope.

The child should be assessed for the degree of dehydration as follows:
- Less than 5% dehydration.
- 5–10% dehydration.
- Greater than 10% dehydration.

In addition, it should be borne in mind that there may be other children at home with diarrhea and vomiting; and that social circumstances may be less than ideal. In these situations admission may be warranted even though the child's condition may not be too severe.

LESS THAN 5% DEHYDRATION

Here the child will be quite well but will exhibit signs of mild dehydration. This will include a dry mouth and lips, and slightly sunken eyes; the child will be awake and alert. Urine output may be decreased and this may be manifest in the form of decreased wetting of nappies. However, this will be difficult to assess if the child has diarrhea.

Treatment consists of oral rehydration with proprietary products. These are often foul tasting, despite attempts at flavoring, due to the high electrolyte content. However, small quantities given regularly may be all that is required to keep the child hydrated. Older children may find it more palatable to eat potato crisps or other proprietary salty snacks and to wash these down with small volumes of electrolyte-poor fluid.

Arrangements should be made for early review of the child, either at home or in the AED, to assess whether he or she is tolerating fluids. Failure to tolerate fluids, or worsening dehydration, should lead one to consider initiating intravenous therapy.

5–10% DEHYDRATION

As fluid loss increases, the child will become progressively more lethargic and the mucous membranes drier (**Figure 3.32**). Small babies may begin to have sunken fontanelles at this stage.

Initially, these children should be admitted for initial oral hydration under medical control. If this measure is

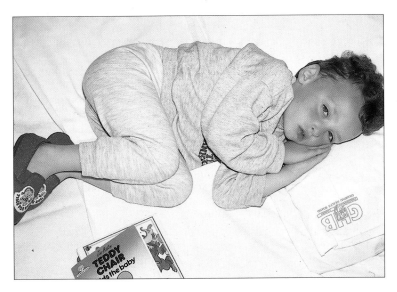

Figure 3.32
Lethargic child with moderate dehydration. Note the sunken eyes, dry lips and general disinterest.

ineffective, then intravenous therapy can be instituted. This will begin with normal saline. Electrolyte analysis will determine whether hypotonic or hypertonic states exist and the fluid therapy altered accordingly.

GREATER THAN 10% DEHYDRATION (SHOCK)

At this level a child will have a significantly altered level of consciousness and may exhibit signs of peripheral shut down (*see* Chapter 1) The child should be treated as would any other child with shock. Airway and breathing should be stabilized and intravenous access established. An initial bolus of 20 ml/kg of normal saline should be administered and the child observed. Further treatment with intravenous rehydration will depend on the response to the initial bolus. The nature of further fluids will also be governed by electrolyte analysis, i.e. hypernatremic or hyponatremic dehydration.

ACUTE POISONING

Acute poisoning can either be accidental or deliberate. Accidental poisoning is usually associated with early childhood with a peak incidence between 2 and 3 years of age. Deliberate poisoning will affect the older age group where it is one of the most common forms of parasuicide. The approach to the initial toxic episode will be similar in both cases, but the after care and follow-up will be different.

The purpose of this section is to give a general approach to the poisoned patient.

More detailed information can be found in a toxicology text book.

In the AED, the doctor should ask the following questions:

- Are the vital signs (**A**irway, **B**reathing and **C**irculation) at risk?
- What substance or combination of substances has the child ingested?
- How much has the child actually ingested?
- What are the potential significant side-effects of the ingested substance(s)?
- If more than one substance has been ingested, what are the potential interactions?
- Is there a specific antidote that should be administered?
- Is gastric decontamination required and how should this be achieved?
- Does the child need admission and, if so, where?
- What follow-up is needed?

VITAL SIGNS

On first seeing the patient, a brief primary survey should be performed (*see* Chapter 1). If the vital functions are at risk appropriate measures should be taken. In some

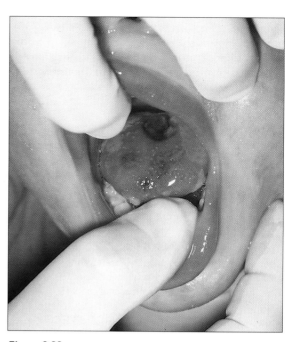

Figure 3.33
Caustic burns to the mouth. This child ingested bleach and sustained significant burns to the airway. Such burns can occur to the pharynx, esophagus and, if aspirated, trachea. This child's airway is at considerable risk.

cases the airway may be safe for a time but will become obstructed if the child is left untreated or unattended. This can happen in cases of caustic ingestion (**Figure 3.33**) and smoke inhalation where the full inflammatory response can take some time to develop. Opiate poisoning treated in the prehospital phase with naloxone can also be dangerous. The half-life of naloxone is only 2 hours but that of opiates is considerably longer. Failure to appreciate this can lead to the respiratory depression and airway obstruction associated with opiate toxicity returning after having been successfully treated previously.

Breathing difficulties can develop some time after aspiration of gastric contents. Iatrogenic aspiration can also occur if gastric lavage or forced emesis is carried out in a child with an inadequately protected airway.

Aspiration of organic compounds such as turpentine or paraffin cause similar delayed respiratory compromise.

Circulatory compromise may be due to:
- Direct myocardial toxicity by the poison.
- Arrhythmias.
- Toxic vasodilation.
- Forced diuresis.
- Blood loss from gastric/intestinal erosions or ulcers.

An altered level of consciousness is common with many poisons. Assessment of the level of consciousness is mandatory as deepening coma will put the airway at risk, lead to respiratory depression and hypoxia and predispose to aspiration. Facilities to protect the airway appropriately should always be to hand (*see* Chapter 1).

WHAT SUBSTANCE OR SUBSTANCES HAVE BEEN INGESTED?

This can be easy to determine if samples of the drug, plant or household product are brought to the AED. Too often, however, one is told it is 'Grannies heart pill' or some such vague statement. Even if samples are to hand plant identification is difficult for non-botanists. The use of books and compter-aided plant identification can help.

Physical signs can also determine the poison (**Figure 3.34**). These can also help track the clinical course of the poisoning episode.

HOW MUCH HAS BEEN INGESTED?

Assessment of the quantity of the poison ingested can be very difficult. A child who opens a bottle of liquid will often spill more down his front or on the floor than he actually ingests. In most cases where pills or capsules are involved, the original quantity is usually unknown.

On the other hand, in the older child who has attempted suicide the actual quantity taken may be deliberately understated in a desperate attempt to obstruct the physician. The amount of absorption of gases or fumes is similarly difficult to quantify. Despite these difficulties every effort should be made to identify the likely quantity involved. In the case of medication, whether over-the-counter or prescribed, it should be possible to estimate the dose per weight taken and relate this to the normal therapeutic dose. The likely toxic effects can then be predicted and hopefully pre-empted.

It is possible to measure serum levels of paracetamol, aspirin and iron. In the case of paracetamol, plasma levels are measured 4 hours after ingestion. Comparison with a nomogram will then determine the likelihood of toxic hepatic damage.

WHAT ARE THE POTENTIAL SIDE-EFFECTS?

It is impossible to know all the possible effects from all possible poisons. For this reason early contact with the local poison's unit is advised as they can give advice on all aspects of treatment. Many areas have a computer-link to the poison's information bureau which can be augmented by clinical advice.

A copy of the poisons advice should be attached to the child's notes, particularly if the child is being admitted. This ensures that all clinicians have access to the same information.

IS THERE AN ANTIDOTE?

The list of potentially useful antidotes is limited. In some cases the antidote or reversing agent is toxic in its own right and so should only be used under guidance of toxicologists (**Figure 3.35**).

GASTRIC DECONTAMINATION

Not every poisoned child needs to undergo gastric decontamination; this is dependent on the substance(s) ingested, the quantity taken, and the likely side-effects. Substances

Pupillary dilation	Tricylic antidepressants
	Atropine
	Sympathomimetic agents
	Belladonna (Foxglove)
	Amphentamines
Pupillary constriction	Opiates
Respiratory depression	Opiates
	Benzodiazepines
	Alcohol
	Phenothiazines
Tachycardia	Tricylic antidepressants
	Atropine
	Sympathomimetic agents
	Aminophylline
Bradycardia	β–Blockers
	Salicylates
Hypotension	Antihypertensive agents
	Tricylic antidepressants
	Calcium channel blockers
	Phenothiazines
Seizure	Tricylic antidepressants
	Mefenamic acid
Coma	Opiates
	Benzodiazepines
	Anticonvulsants
	Alcohol
Agitation	Cannabis
	Alcohol
	Metaclopramide

Figure 3.34

Some common features associated with poisoning and common causative agents. The list is not exhaustive and if there is concern, a poisons information centre should be contacted.

Figure 3.35

Some antidotes to various poisons

Poison	Antidote	Comments
Opiates	Naloxone	Half-life <2 hours which is usually greater than that of ingested opiate
β-blockers	Glucagon Isoprenaline	Need cardiac monitoring
Benzodiazepines	Flumazanil	Should not be used if multiple drugs involved. Routine use discouraged
Paracetamol (acetaminophen)	N-Acetylcysteine or Methionine	Methionine can cause vomiting as can paracetamol IV treatment can be difficult as fluid volumes high for small children
Phenothiazine or Metaclopramide	Procyclidine	
Tricyclic anti-depressant	Physostigmine Bicarbonate	May aggravate cardiac toxicity. Not routinely advocated
Digoxin	'FAB' antibodies	Discuss with poison's bureau before use
Iron	Desferrioxamine	Discuss with poison's bureau before use Consider NG dosage as well as IM
Cyanide	Kelocyanor or 'Cyanide kit'	Kelocyanor toxic in the absence of cyanide toxicity! Use only in cardiac arrest due to cyanide

such as antibiotics, soap, liquid mercury (**not mercuric salts**) and vitamins without iron are all benign. A full list of non-toxic substances can be found in any standard text on poisons.

Forced gastric emptying is a very unpleasant process and distressing for all concerned. It should never be undertaken as a punishment. The young child is usually unaware that a wrong has been committed and the depressed adolescent is unlikely to be deterred from further over-doses unless the underlying illness or aggravating factors are removed.

The practice of forced gastric emptying has been called into question in any case. The use of charcoal has been increasingly advocated. However, it is not always easy to persuade a small child to voluntarily drink a glass of charcoal!

Gastric lavage (**Figure 3.36**) should be undertaken in the following circumstances:

- The substances involved are likely to have a prolonged effect if not actively removed, for example, gastric erosions from salicylate.
- Emesis is not advised due to the airway being potentially or actually at risk (for example unconscious).
- If charcoal or other antidotes (for example desferrioxamine) need to be left in the stomach.

Before gastric lavage is performed the child should be assessed with regard to the level of consciousness and the potential for the poison to cause coma. If there is any risk to the airway the child should be electively anesthetized and intubated.

Care must be taken that potential anesthetic agents do not interact adversely with the poison, particularly with regard to cardiotoxicity.

The child should be placed in the left lateral position and a large-bore nasogastric tube passed into the stomach. Aspiration of gastric contents will confirm correct placement, as will testing the aspirate with litmus paper (it should show an acid response). As much of the gastric contents as possible should be aspirated using a syringe. Thereafter, aliquots of water should be instilled and aspirated until no particulate matter is withdrawn. At this stage charcoal or other antidotes can be instilled down the tube and left *in situ*. Care must be taken with charcoal. Reports exist of semicomatose persons with inadequately protected airways aspirating charcoal with resultant pneumonitis.

Forced emesis may be undertaken using syrup of ipecacuanha. Doses of 15–30 ml can be given according to age. Emesis usually occurs within 30 minutes and can be aided by placing the child on a rocking horse! It is most effective when given soon after the poisoning; particularly within 1 hour of poisoning. However routine use is diminishing in favour of charcoal.

CHARCOAL (Figure 3.37)

In many cases, charcoal is increasingly advocated as an alternative to emesis. It acts by adsorbing the toxic substances in the gastrointestinal tract and so reduces absorption. However, it can be difficult to persuade the child to take the dose prescribed!

ADMISSION

Most cases of poisoning can be managed on an outpatient basis. Indications to admit include:

- Coma or potential alteration of consciousness.
- Existing airway distress, aspiration or potential for respiratory compromise.
- Circulatory collapse.

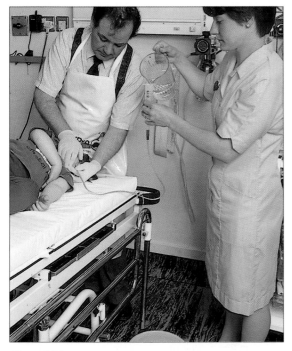

Figure 3.36
Gastric lavage. This should not be undertaken in a comatose child unless the airway is fully protected.

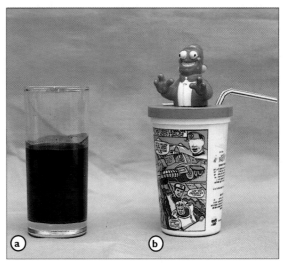

Figure 3.37
The appearance of charcoal in a glass makes it unappealing for a child to take. Charcoal in a glass (a) and in a fun container (b) where the child can drink it unseen through a straw.

- Cardiac arrhythmias.
- Convulsions.
- Metabolic or electrolyte disturbances.
- Further treatment needed, for example, *N*-acetylcysteine in paracetamol poisoning.
- Possible delayed effects of the drug, for example, gastric/intestinal erosions in iron poisoning.
- Concern about the safety of the child, for example, serious suicide risk or at risk of child abuse.

FOLLOW-UP ARRANGEMENTS

Accidental poisoning, particularly in the younger age group, may be a harbinger of family stress or neglect. It should alert the community services to the need for a follow-up appointment, either by a health visitor or the family physician. Stress, poor family dynamics or other risk factors can be explored either formally or informally. An assessment of the further risk of poisoning or other accident can then be made and possible preventive measures advised.

Children who deliberately ingest poisons as a parasuicide or a 'cry for help' should be referred to the appropriate social or psychiatric services. Different health authorities will have different policies.

Poisoning from alcohol, glue sniffing or experimentation with illegal drugs poses a difficult dilemma. Many children go through a phase of peer-group experimentation, which can be regarded as a 'normal' learning process. This may be best dealt with by educational programs in the community. However, abuse of these substances in isolation as a singular activity should be regarded as pathological and should receive more serious attention.

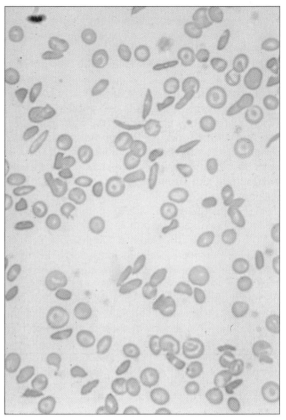

Figure 3.38
Child with sickle cell trait. Note the crescent-shaped cells which cause all the problems.

HEMATOLOGY

Hematology problems are infrequent in the AED. Several conditions deserve a mention. These include:
- Anemia.
- Sickle cell disease.
- Bleeding disorders.
- Leukemia.

ANEMIA

The causes of anemia in children are many, but, as with most things in medicine, only a few present with regularity. Most children who are anemic are iron deficient, usually due to a poor dietary intake. If such a deficiency is suspected, serum iron should be measured and oral supplements of iron started. A repeat blood count should be carried out after 7–10 days. Failure to see an improvement with therapy is an indication for specialist referral.

SICKLE CELL DISEASE (Figure 3.38)

This disorder primarily affects those of Afro–Caribbean extraction. It is inherited in an autosomal recessive manner. Affected children are prone to sickle-cell crises during acute febrile illness, particularly those causing hypoxia and dehydration.

Children with sickle cell disease are prone to infections which in turn aggravate the disease. Complications associated with crises include anemia and infarction.

Children with sickle cell disease usually have a low hemoglobin count but during the crisis there may be increased hemolysis and an associated failure of the marrow to generate new red blood cells. Typically, there will be a hemolytic blood picture without a concomitant rise in circulating reticulocytes.

During a sickle-cell crisis pain is a significant feature. This is due to infarction, especially in bone. This is due to increased viscosity in the microvascular system, caused by the lack of deformability of red corpuscles. This is aggravated by dehydration.

While bone infarcts are commonest, any end-organ can be affected, including the brain (leading to cerebral infarction) and the eye (retinal artery thrombosis).

The general principles of resuscitation apply. In addition, analgesia is needed if there is evidence of infarction or bone pain. Consideration should be given for antibiotic-treatment if infectious disease is thought to be present.

Sickle cell trait, in which the amount of sickle-cell hemoglobin (HbS) is very much less, is not associated with the extremes of illness present in the full-blown disease. However, severe infection, especially if associated with hypoxia, may lead to problems similar to that described above.

BLEEDING DISORDERS

Children with inherited or acquired bleeding disorders are usually well known to the Hematology Service. Consequently, they rarely present to the AED for routine treatment of acute bleeds. If they do, early contact with the Hematology Service is mandatory. This is especially true if the child presents with a lesion, such as a wound or fracture, which may need additional clotting factor cover before any procedure is carried out.

Children can present *de novo* with a purpuric rash of 2–3 days' duration. The differential diagnosis is large but platelet disorders need to be excluded. Including idiopathic thromobocytopenic purpura. (**Figure 3.39**). Leukemia (*see* next section) and other marrow suppressive disorders need to be excluded. Referral to a hematologist is advised for further evaluation of the problem.

Bleeding disorders due to deficiencies in clotting factors occasionally present to the AED. There may be persistent bleeding following dental extraction or repair of

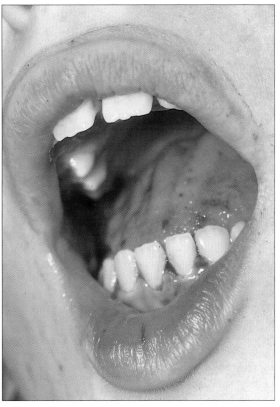

Figure 3.39
Idiopathic thrombocytopenic purpura. Intra-oral purpuric lesions with bleeding around the gum margins.

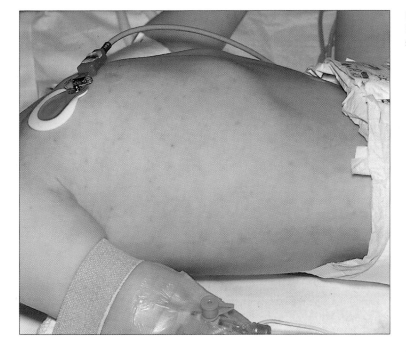

Figure 3.40
Purpuric rash with meningococcal septicemia.

a minor wound. Occasionally, children will be referred as 'possible non-accidental injury' (*see* Chapter 4) due to bruising being present. Even more rarely children will present with complications from an intracranial hematoma.

If a bleeding disorder is suspected, a full clotting screen, full blood count and film and a platelet count should be requested. Any abnormality found should be discussed with a hematologist.

LEUKEMIA

Children with leukemia can present to the AED under a number of guises and with misleading symptoms. These include limp, hip pain, bone pain, malaise, anemia and abdominal pain among others (see Chapter 5).

If leukemia is suspected, a blood film should be sent to the laboratory for examination by a hematologist. If the diagnosis is confirmed the child should be referred as an emergency to a specialist service.

THE UNWELL CHILD

This is a common presentation of children in AEDs, particularly for those in the first few years of life. Broadly speaking, these children can be grouped into three categories:
- Less than 3 months of age.
- Three months to 3 years of age.
- Over 3 years of age.

CHILDREN 0–3 MONTHS OF AGE

These children appear frequently in the AED. They either self-present or are referred by the family doctor for further assessment and management.

Typically, their history is vague. Diffuse symptoms such as possible apneic attacks, off feeds, vomiting or mother reporting the child is 'not well' are frequent. In these children, sepsis, occult or florid, should be uppermost in the mind. Other causes include cardiac failure, supraventricular tachycardia (SVT) and inborn errors of metabolism. These children, even if septic, will not necessarily be pyrexial and even a white cell count can be normal.

It is incumbent on every doctor in these situations to perform a full physical examination looking for a focus of infection. This will include upper respiratory tract, chest and urinary tract infections together with meningitis. Occult causes such as appendicitis and osteomyelitis also have to be considered as will surgical causes, for example, obstructed inguinal hernia. Intussusception and appendicitis are rare but need to be considered. If no obvious cause for the problem is found the child should be admitted for further observation. A septic screen may be indicated.

A decision to start or withhold antibiotics in this situation is clinically difficult and will rely on the condition of the child and the expertise/seniority of the admitting physicians. If in doubt, a broad spectrum antibiotic such as ceftriaxone will adequately provide antimicrobial cover for most septic causes.

Children who have a focus for infection in this age group and who have sufficient symptomatology for them to present to an AED should be taken seriously. It is probably preferable to admit these children even for a short period of time to assess progress in response to treatment.

CHILDREN 3 MONTHS TO 3 YEARS OF AGE

These form one of the larger cohorts of the AED. Most will have an underlying viral illness. Focal bacterial infection or bacteremia are also important causes. The distinction between viral and bacterial focal infections becomes easier as the child gets older.

Typically, viral infections will have multiple mucous membrane involvement, for example, watery eyes, running nose, red ears and red throat. Bacterial infections tend to affect one area only. In a number of cases no focal source will be found for the infection and in these situations the differences between bacteremia and occult infection, such as meningitis, septic arthritis and osteomyelitis, can be difficult to spot.

Pointers include the level of the temperature and the level of the white blood cell count. A white cell count greater than 15 000 per μl, particularly with a neutrophil differential and a temperature of 39°C or above, is strongly indicative of significant bacterial infection. In patients with temperatures of less than 39°C and white cell counts of <10 000 per μl it is unlikely that any significant bacterial infection is present. White cell counts of less than 5000 per μl can be found in severely septic children, so these parameters need to be assessed in the context of the entire clinical picture.

Other features which raise concern about the underlying problem include the presence of petechial rash or circulatory compromise (*see* Chapter 1). In these situations, significant bacterial infection should be considered and treated accordingly (**Figure 3.41**).

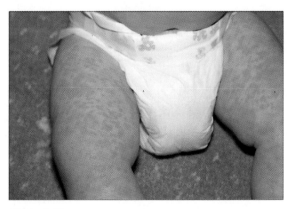

Figure 3.41
Typical maculopapular viral rash over a child's lower limb.

Surgical conditions, for example, obstructed hernia, intussusception and appendicitis also need to be considered (*see* Chapter 5).

MANAGEMENT

A full physical examination should be performed looking for focal signs of infection. A septic screen should be done which may or may not include lumbar puncture. Certainly, the closer a child is to the neonatal period the lower the threshold should be for a lumbar puncture.

Outpatient therapy can be considered if there is a single focal infection, the child is not toxic, home circumstances are good, and early follow-up can be obtained. Otherwise, it is prudent to admit the child for a period of inpatient therapy. The treatment of likely causes is included under the relevant diagnostic headings earlier in this chapter.

Of particular relevance, however, is the need to follow-up urinary tract infections that can lead to renal tract damage if not treated appropriately.

CHILDREN OVER 3 YEARS OF AGE

Focal bacterial infections occur less frequently in this age group although they are by no means unknown. Typically, these children are more articulate and able to communicate more easily than younger children. They are able to give better descriptions of symptoms and signs are easier to elicit. The same general principles of treatment apply in so far as toxic children without a focus of infection should probably be admitted and intravenous antibiotics can be considered. Those with focal infection which is obvious and amenable to treatment should be allowed home for outpatient treatment and early follow-up.

DERMATOLOGIC MANIFESTATIONS OF SYSTEMIC DISEASE

There are a number of dermatologic conditions that are associated with underlying systemic disease. Often no underlying diagnosis or predisposing cause will be found.

RASHES

Children often present with erythematous maculopapular rashes (**Figure 3.41**). The rash may occur 2–3 days after the onset of conditions such as coryza, inflamed ears and throat. Often the parents are unconcerned about the symptoms and only become aware when the rash appears. It is important to distinguish a maculopapular rash from a purpuric rash, the latter often being associated with significant systemic disease; **a maculopapular rash will blanche on pressure whereas a purpuric rash will not**.

ERYTHEMA MULTIFORME

Erythema multiforme is a form of allergic reaction, usually to viral infection or mycopcasma (**Figure 3.42**). Typically, there are raised erythematous margins with a central pale area (target lesion). It can range from a mild rash to a breakdown of mucous membranes as in Stevens–Johnson syndrome.

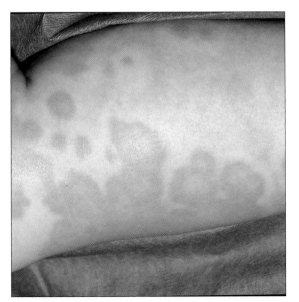

Figure 3.42
Erythema multiforme. Note the target lesions with central white areas surround by red, raised, erythematous areas.

ERYTHEMA NODOSUM

This lesion follows streptococcal infections, viral infections and occasionally tuberculosis. Painful raised erythematous lesions are present on the anterior of the shins (**Figure 3.43**).

HENOCH–SCHÖNLEIN PURPURA

This is a disease of unknown etiology. It can be multisystemic in nature with renal, gastrointestinal and synovial involvement added to the skin manifestations (**Figure 3.44 a**). Renal involvement can include hematuria, proteinuria and nephritis. Gastrointestinal tract involvement can manifest as abdominal pain. A small number of patients will develop intussusception. A mucosal vasculitis can lead to melena. Joint pains and effusions can also occur.

Typically, the skin exhibits a purpuric rash on the extensor surfaces (**Figure 3.44 b**).

Unless complications are present the child can be managed expectantly.

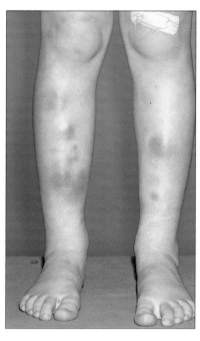

Figure 3.43
Erythema nodosum. Note the red, raised lesions over the right shin. It is easy to confuse these with bruises which might be sustained during a football match.

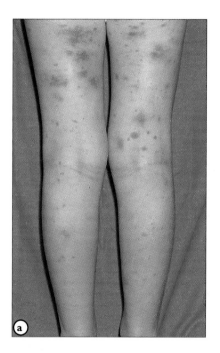

Figure 3.44 a
Purpuric rash over the extensor surface typical of Henoch–Schönlein purpura.

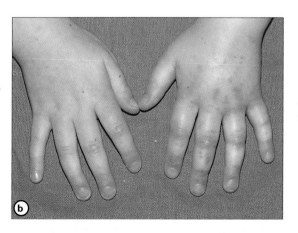

Figure 3.44 b
Henoch–Schönlein purpura with arthritis. Note the swelling of the left hand and wrist with associated purpuric lesions.

Chapter FOUR

Pediatric Trauma

Accidents and other trauma are the leading cause of death in childhood. Road Traffic Accidents (RTAs) are the most common cause in the UK with 55% of all deaths occuring as a result. Of the remainder, most die in their homes from burns, scalds, falls and other incidents.

Accident prevention initiaives have an important role to play in reducing morbidity and mortality. These will take time and effort to have maximal effect, and the role of the AED in such initiatives must not be underestimated (Chapter 1).

Until these initiatives begin to take effect there will be a need for effective care of the severely injured child.

APPROACH TO THE MANAGEMENT OF THE SEVERELY INJURED CHILD

As with all resuscitation sequences, the child should be approached in a logical and constructive manner. It is helpful to subdivide this approach into the following areas:
- Primary survey.
- Definitive resuscitation.
- Secondary survey.
- Discharge/transfer.

PRIMARY SURVEY

The priority in the primary survey is to identify any immediate life-threatening condition. This will involve rapid assessment of the airway, breathing, circulation, and disability.

AIRWAY CARE

When dealing with the airway in the injured child, it is important not to move the neck any more than is absolutely necessary. Ideally, the airway should be opened with the head immobilized completely; no rotation, or extension/flexion should be allowed of the cervical spine. Therefore the method of choice in opening the airway should be by chin lift **only** (as opposed to chin lift and head tilt).

Gentle suction may be needed to clear blood, vomitus or secretions from the pharynx.

Children are prone to a condition called Spinal Cord Injury Without Radiologic Abnormality (SCIWORA) (**Figure 4.1**). This condition is particularly important in children who are unconscious. In this syndrome, the spinal cord may be traumatised even though no abnormality can be seen on plain X-rays. The worry is that a partial spinal cord injury may be present and that by failing to immo-

bilize the cervical spine it could be converted to complete spinal cord damage.

Because the condition cannot be diagnosed radiologically, all unconscious children should be treated as having a SCIWORA until such time as the integrity of the spinal cord can be established either clinically or radiologically.

If intubation is needed then the head must not be flexed on the spine. Inline traction should be maintained to avoid

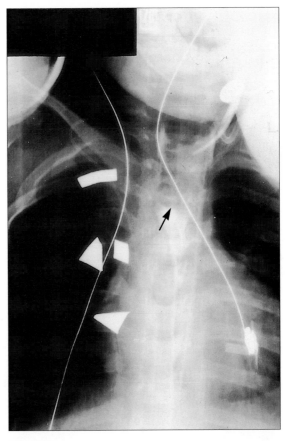

Figure 4.1
SCIWORA: myelogram demonstrating no contrast above the level of D4 (arrow). This child had no bony abnormality on either plain radiograph or computerized tomography (CT) imaging. He is paralysed from D4 down.

this. Similarly, if bag/valve/mask ventilation is required care must be taken to avoid moving the neck (**Figure 4.2**).

SPINAL IMMOBILIZATION
Cervical spine immobilization
This is best achieved by the application of a firm collar that reduces flexion/extension movements in the neck. Lateral movement is discouraged by applying blanket rolls to the side of the head. These should then be taped in place (**Figure 4.3**).

Protection of the dorsal and lumbar spine
This is achieved by keeping the child flat and avoiding any flexion/extension movements. Later in the resuscitation process it will be necessary to move the child to examine the back. This will be described at a later point in this chapter (**Figures 4.12a and b**)

BREATHING
Once the airway is open the efficiency of breathing should be established. In the first instance, if the child is no breath-ing or breathing efforts are inadequate bag/valve/mask ventilation should be established. Underlying causes of the child's difficulty in breathing should be diagnosed and treated. The underlying causes of breathing difficulties include:

- Airway obstruction—perform airway-opening maneuvers again, consider a foreign body (including secretions) (*see* Chapter 1).
- Pneumothorax—listen over both lung fields with a stethoscope, and use needle thoracostomy if pneumothorax is present (*see* Chapter 1).
- Gastric dilatation—insert a large-bore gastric tube and decompress the stomach (*see* **Figure 4.9,4.82**).

CIRCULATION
The efficacy of the circulation should be assessed as described in Chapter 1. In addition, any obvious bleeding points that can be easily controlled using external pressure should be attended to. This is not the time to begin treatment of minor wounds; these can be dealt with when the patient is stable and out of danger. Intravenous cannulae should be inserted and fluid replacement commenced according to the clinical state. A bolus of 20 ml/kg of normal saline is appropriate initially.

DISABILITY
Disability relates primarily to the level of consciousness and, at later stages to the assessment of the full neurologic status of the patient. As discussed in the chapter on cardiac arrest (*see* Chapter 2), any alteration in the level of consciousness predisposes to airway obstruction. It takes time to perform a full Glasgow Coma Scale assessment and initially it is better to do a brief informal assessment. One available scale is the AVPU scale (*see* Chapter 1, **Figure 1.56**). This will allow a working diagnosis of the level of consciousness to be made and the appropriate action to be taken.

An altered level of consciousness may be due to hypovolemia and/or hypoxia. These should be corrected and a further assessment made.

Pupillary reactions can be assessed at this stage.

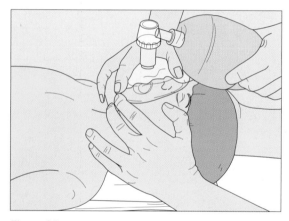

Figure 4.2
Inline traction must be maintained to minimize and hopefully prevent flexion, extension movements, and left or right movement of the cervical spine, even while ventilatory procedures are being carried out.

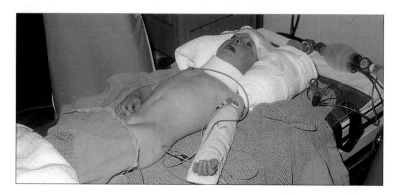

Figure 4.3
A traumatized child immobilized with blanket rolls and tape and a soft cervical collar. Intravenous access has been established and he has been undressed to facilitate a secondary survey. It is important to make sure that he is kept warm.

DEFINITIVE RESUSCITATION

Definitive resuscitation involves securing an airway permanently, controlling ventilation (including formal chest drainage), and controlling hemorrhage. The latter may require transfer of the child to the operating theatre and takes precedence over all other procedures. Appropriate fluid-replacement therapy should be continued.

Part of the resuscitation will involve giving the child adequate analgesia, splinting all limbs that are obviously broken, and insertion of tubes into the stomach and the bladder.

ANALGESIA

Analgesia is often withheld unnecessarily in children who have been traumatized. The major problem is with children who have had a minor head injury and who have orthopedic problems. However, children who have chest/abdominal trauma may also be in pain and providing analgesia may make assessment easier. Several methods of analgesia are available:

- Opiate analgesia, either intramuscularly or intravenously.
- Diclofenac/codeine phosphate, intramuscularly.
- Local nerve block.
- Oral analgesia.
- Inhalation analgesia.
- Splinting.

Children who have an altered level of consciousness and who require surgery are usually rapidly anesthetized and analgesics given. In this situation, pain relief is given as part of the anesthesia.

Intravenous opiates

This is probably the route of choice for all children with orthopedic trauma. Our preference is to use morphine at the following doses:

1. less than 1 year of age,   0.1 mg/kg.
2. more than 1 year of age, 0.2 mg/kg.

Small babies have a reduced ability to metabolize opiates and therefore there is a greater chance of overdosage if the lower dose is not used.

To give analgesia, the recommended dosage should be drawn up and then diluted to 10 ml. One can administer a 3 ml bolus and titrate 1 ml/minute until analgesia is established. Very often only half the dose is required initially but this may need to be topped up at regular intervals. This method of opiate administration has many benefits. Firstly, it avoids over-rapid infusion thus obviating respiratory embarrassment and vomiting. Secondly, given in this fashion it has minimal effect on the level of consciousness. Thirdly, the analgesia reaches the circulation reliably.

Intramuscular opiates are not recommended (*see* next section).

Intramuscular diclofenac/codine phosphate

Diclofenac is being used more frequently in the trauma-tized child. It has the advantage of not reducing the level of consciousness and does not interfere with head injury observation. Codeine phosphate is also widely used.

The disadvantage of these drugs is that they are administered intramuscularly which makes their use painful for the child undergoing treatment; their absorption from intramuscular sites is also unreliable. Diclofenac itself, by any route, will have a tendency to cause gastric erosions.

Local nerve block (Figures 4.4 and 4.5)

There is no doubt that local anesthesia, using prilocaine, lignocaine or bupivacaine, is effective in reducing pain from a fracture; it makes the child more comfortable and, if possible, should be used in preference to other forms of analgesia.

Oral analgesia

There is no place for oral medication in major trauma.

Inhalation analgesia

Mixtures of nitrous oxide and oxygen are readily available. They should not be used in children who are suspected of having a pneumothorax. Inhalation analgesia may help with some procedures, such as application of a long leg cast, if local nerve block cannot be obtained.

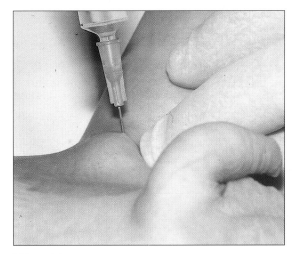

Figure 4.4
Femoral nerve block.

Sites for local nerve block	
Fracture site	**Injection**
Femur	Femoral nerve block
Tibia	Sciatic nerve block
Humerus	Scalene nerve block
Rib	Intercostal nerve block

Figure 4.5

Splinting

Other measures to reduce pain include the application of appropriate splints. Unfortunately, very few splints are available for children. As discussed previously, children come in all shapes and sizes and trying to match the splint to the child is an extremely difficult exercise (**Figures 4.6–4.8**).

GASTRIC TUBES (Figure 4.9)

Gastric tubes should be inserted via the mouth if there is any suspicion of a base-of-skull fracture—they will rapidly decompress the stomach which tends to undergo dilata-

tion in a traumatized child. Why this happens is unclear. There is no doubt that many children get significant relief from drainage of gastric contents. This will relieve pressure on the diaphragm and very often results in adequate respiration and ventilation being established. It also renders the abdomen easier to examine (*see* **Figure 4.9**, **Figure 4.82**).

URINARY CATHETERS

Urinary catheters are useful in shocked and unconscious children. They relieve the pain of a distended bladder and

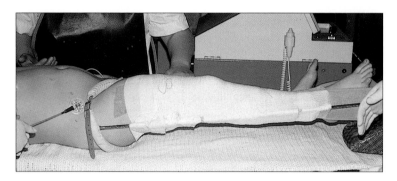

Figure 4.6
Thomas splint in place for a fracture of the midshaft of the right femur. Care must be taken that the circular support around the groin does not get too tight.

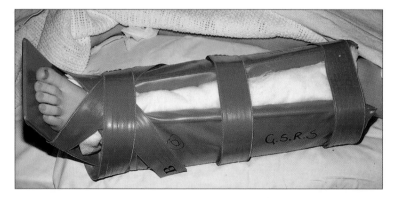

Figure 4.7.
Commercialy available box splint for immobilizing a fractured tibia. This will not be suitable for younger children as it is too big.

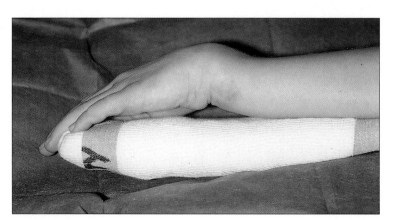

Figure 4.8
Fracture of the distal radius and ulna with angulation. A 'homemade' splint has been prepared and this will be held in place with a bandage prior to the child going to X-ray. Analgesia has already been administered.

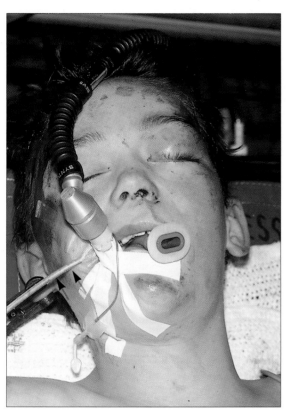

Figure 4.9
A young male with significant head injury sustained in a road traffic accident. Clinically, he has a basal skull fracture suspected as a result of bruising to the left eye and blood coming from the left nostril. A gastric tube (arrowed) has been passed and is draining gastric contents. Nasal tubes are contra indicated.(see text). As an aside a cuffed ETT has been passed but the cuff is not inflated.

enable accurate measurements of urine output. In burned or shocked children a urinary output of between 1 and 2 ml/kg/hour should be achieved. Any persistent fall below 1 ml/kg/hour should lead to a suspicion that the child is underperfused.

HISTORY

Following stabilization of the child it is important to speak to anyone who may have been at the scene of the accident—this will include ambulance staff, police, firemen and relatives. The ambulance staff are likely to be more objective in the history than relatives or other witnesses. The following questions should be asked:

1. What safety equipment was being used, for example, helmet, safety belts (**Figure 4.10**)?
2. What damage was done to these and were they effective in limiting injury?
3. How close to the vehicle or the incident was the child found?
4. In what condition was the child at the scene?
5. What resuscitation and other treatment was needed *en route*?

A further aspect of the history is to find out as much as possible about the child that is relevant to his or her current state; this will often only be available if the parents are present (**Figure 4.11**).

SECONDARY SURVEY

The secondary survey begins with a full neurologic examination. It is at this stage that a full assessment of the child's level of consciousness may be made. Unfortunately, this is often compromised by the fact that the child has had to be paralyzed and ventilated prior to the neurologic examination. If

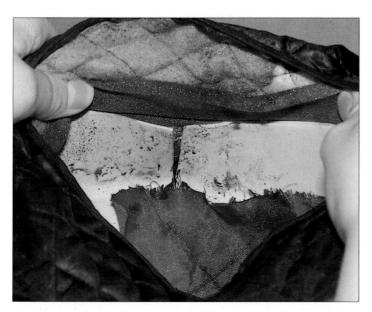

Figure 4.10
The riding hat of a child thrown from her horse. The horse was seen to kick the child's head and had she not been wearing the helmet the fracture shown would have been present in the child's skull. A history of damage to protective devices should always be taken and is a good assessment of the force applied.

Extra history for traumatised children	
L	Last ate or drank
A	Allergies
M	Medication
P	Past medical history

Figure 4.11

at all possible, a full neurologic assessment should be conducted before the child has been fully sedated to enable determination of full neurologic signs, differences in muscle strength (allowing for the presence of fractures), and the state of the reflexes. Symmetry can also be assessed.

Neurologic examination should be followed by thorough palpation of every bone in the body. A full examination of the ears, mouth, and nose should be made to look for evidence of a base-of-skull fracture manifested by blood or cerebrospinal fluid (CSF) leakage.

The chest should be examined thoroughly, both front and back, using a log-roll if neccesary (**Figure 4.12a and b**). The abdomen should be palpated carefully. Great care should be taken to examine the scrotum in males and the urethra in both males and females to ensure that no lacerations are present and there is no blood at the meatus in the male.

If possible, a rectal examination should be carried out at this stage with the child on his/her back. Particular care should be taken to assess anal sphincter tone and the patency of reflexes around the perineum.

It is then prudent to log-roll the child with full spinal precautions to examine the back and remove clothing.

LOG-ROLL (Figure 4.12a and b)

It is important to turn the child onto their side to examine the back for the following reasons:

- To inspect the back and examine the spinal column.
- To remove clothing and wet blankets that may be present.
- To remove any foreign bodies or debris that may have accumulated prior to the child being rescued.

When performing a log-roll it is important that the neck is kept immobilized and that it is not rotated on the dorsal spine. Similarly, it is important that the dorsal spine and lumbar spine do not rotate or flex/extend.

To perform a log-roll a minimum of four people are needed. One person is designated to control the head and neck. Two people control the chest, abdomen, pelvis and legs; a third person will be needed to assist with this in older children and adolescents. An additional person is designated to examine the spine and remove clothing and debris once the child has been turned.

Once the child has been rolled and all the necessary procedures carried out he or she is laid back, again in one piece without any rotation.

Once physical examination is complete, appropriate X-rays are taken. In a child with multiple injuries it is mandatory to examine the the cervical spine, chest, abdomen and pelvis.

A decision is made as to where the X-rays are taken. If X-ray equipment is installed in the resuscitation room there is no problem. If there is only portable equipment

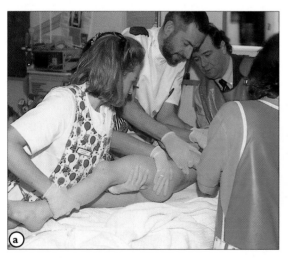

Figure 4.12 a

Log-roll. The purpose of a log-roll is to enable a child to be moved onto his/her side for detailed examination of the back. It is important that it is done in a controlled manner with somebody detailed to look after the airway and cervical spine. Extra people are needed to rotate the trunk and pelvis and an extra person is required to allow for any fractured limbs which need to be splinted. A doctor should be available on the side facing the back, once the child has been log-rolled, to ensure that a detailed examination of the spine and rectum takes place.

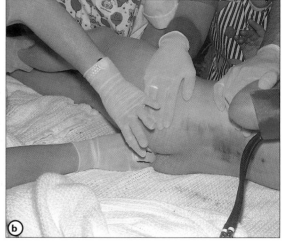

Figure 4.12 b

This child has been log-rolled using several pairs of hands to ensure in line movement. A doctor has been allocated to examine the exposed dorsal surface. This demonstrates the importance of log-rolling a child where significant abrasions are noted over the left renal area. The doctor is examining the anal region to assess anal tone.

available in the resuscitation room then there is a trade-off between film quality and safety of the patient. Certainly no unstable patient should leave the resuscitation room for radiologic examination that will not alter management.

If X-rays are taken in the resuscitation room, portable or otherwise, the radiation protection rules of the hospital must be observed and no one person should be regularly exposed to radiation.

It is desirable to request X-rays according to the injuries detected during physical examination. However, the broad principle 'that if a bone is bent it is broken' should hold. This means one should not wait for X-rays of the affected parts to be carried out while life-threatening conditions are present.

There is debate as to whether or not plain X-rays should be taken of the skull in this situation. If the child requires a CT scan it is unnecessary to perform plain-skull X-rays.

Additional imaging of the abdomen may be necessary (**Figure 4.13**). Where available, ultrasound can be a useful tool in experienced hands. Free fluid and organ damage can be detected. Where ultrasound or experienced radiologists are not available, a CT scan may be performed. CT is more sensitive in bowel rupture, pancreatic damage and skeletal abnormality, detecting and demonstrating multiple visceral injury. It is accepted that ultrasound is a helpful first line of investigation. Being portable it can be transported to the resuscitation room where the child can be examined during resuscitation.

Free fluid in the abdomen without obvious organ damage should lead one to consider laparotomy, as the incidence of bowel perforation and other such injuries is high. If the abdominal examination reveals organ damage, a decision will have to be made by the surgical team as to whether operation is indicated (*see* Abdominal trauma).

It is prudent to carry out a full blood count, analyze urea and electrolyte levels, and send blood for group and cross match when intravenous lines are erected. If pancreatic trauma is suspected then a serum amylase assay is helpful.

BLOOD TESTS

It is not always possible to obtain as much blood from a child as one would wish. However, certain tests are mandatory in trauma and these should always be performed (**Figure 4.14**). If sufficient blood is left over then further analyses may be performed as required. In a critically injured child, arterial blood should always be analyzed for blood gases.

DISPOSAL/TRANSFER

Hopefully by now a comprehensive well coordinated review of the child's condition will have been made. Airway, breathing and circulation should all have been stabilized. Clinical examination allied to radiological and hematologic investigation should give a good idea of the underlying injuries present.

A decision now has to be made regarding the most suitable transfer destination for the child. This will obviously depend on the nature of the institution to which the child has been admitted. Many children will be able to remain in low-level institutions but those with head, chest and abdominal injuries who require surgery, and orthopedic injuries requiring complex orthopedic and plastic surgical assessment, will need to be transferred to specialist units.

Even if the child has been admitted to a recognized trauma center and subsequent transfer is only in-house from the resuscitation room to either radiology or the wards, similar procedures for transferring the child should be in place.

Patient transfer is not the role of junior members of staff.

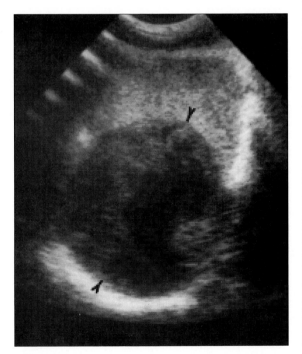

Figure 4.13
Sagittal ultrasound section through the spleen. The small arrows indicate a splenic hematoma.

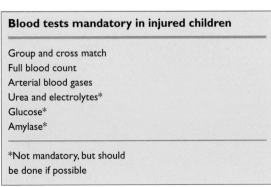

Blood tests mandatory in injured children
Group and cross match
Full blood count
Arterial blood gases
Urea and electrolytes*
Glucose*
Amylase*
*Not mandatory, but should be done if possible

Figure 4.14

Prior to transfer, it is important to have a checklist of all the important features that need to be dealt with.

Particular care should be taken with the airway, breathing, and circulation. If the child has been intubated, it is important that experienced staff accompany the child during transfer. Prior to departure the endotracheal tube should be checked for length and patency. Correct ventilation in both lung fields should be ensured. Adequate means to ventilate the child should be available. Any chest drain should be carefully monitored. It is important not to raise an underwater seal above the level of the chest; this will result in siphoning of fluid into the chest.

All gastric tubes, urinary catheters, and drainage bags should be secured. If the child has been paralyzed and ventilated it is important to bring sufficient drugs to top-up the anesthesia. If portable syringe drivers are being used it is important that spare batteries are available.

Adequate monitoring equipment should be available. At the very least a functioning pulse oximeter with adequate battery life should be available.

All documentation relating to the child should be taken with the child when he or she is transferred. This will include X-rays, results of blood tests, and all clinical details. Personnel skilled in reintubation and airway care should accompany the child. Similarly, a nurse should be available who is proficient in assisting in all aspects of resuscitation care. If parents are unable to accompany the child, written consent for further emergency procedures should be obtained and sent with the child.

POSTRESUSCITATION

Staff who are left behind must replenish all stocks and ensure that everything is in order, ready for the next resuscitation. All equipment that has been used should be checked and replaced with working equipment.

If the child has died within the AED, the general practitioner will need to be notified as will the health visitor and the legal authorities.

DEBRIEFING

If possible a debriefing and audit of the resuscitation should be carried out as soon as possible after the event.

ORGANIZATION OF TRAUMA RESUSCITATION (Figure 4.15)

Trauma resuscitation, like attendance at cardiac arrest, needs to be structured and organized. One method of organizing and deploying staff appears on the accompanying chart (**Figure 4.15**). Again, as in the treatment of cardiac arrest (*see* Chapter 2), Doctor 1 has overall responsibility for the care of the patient, together with simple measures to maintain the airway. This doctor should be capable of definitive airway care should the need arise. It is this doctor's responsibility to ensure that there is no neck movement or spinal rotation until such time as it is confirmed that the spine is uninjured.

Two I.V. lines should be inserted if at all possible. Usually fluid is only delivered through one line in the first instance, but in a severely ill child the second line may be required. Once intravenous access is obtained blood samples should be taken, as previously detailed, and sent to the laboratory. Doctor 2 should take responsibility for this while Doctor 3 begins a complete secondary survey. Any life-threatening or potentially life-threatening injuries detected at this stage should be treated in a definitive

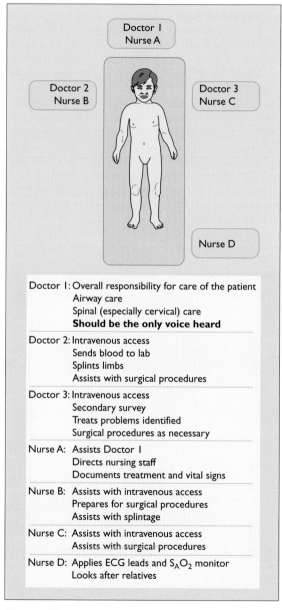

Doctor 1:	Overall responsibility for care of the patient Airway care Spinal (especially cervical) care **Should be the only voice heard**
Doctor 2:	Intravenous access Sends blood to lab Splints limbs Assists with surgical procedures
Doctor 3:	Intravenous access Secondary survey Treats problems identified Surgical procedures as necessary
Nurse A:	Assists Doctor 1 Directs nursing staff Documents treatment and vital signs
Nurse B:	Assists with intravenous access Prepares for surgical procedures Assists with splintage
Nurse C:	Assists with intravenous access Assists with surgical procedures
Nurse D:	Applies ECG leads and S_AO_2 monitor Looks after relatives

Figure 4.15
Suggested organization and duties of staff for trauma resuscitation (see main text for further details).

manner prior to going on to the next stage. Injuries detected at this stage may include pneumothorax, gastric dilatation, abdominal problems, and absent pulses secondary to fractures.

Nursing staff should be directed to assist with all of these procedures. It is imperative that one nurse be detailed to monitor fluid therapy as it is easy for over transfusion to take place if care is not taken to measure the volumes of fluid administered. Similarly, once fluids have been given, the cannula should be heparinized if no further fluid is needed.

It is important to make sure that relatives are well looked after and comforted appropriately. Once resuscitation is well under way they may be able to attend to their child, but only if their presence does not interfere with the resuscitation process.

HEAD INJURY

Head injury is one of the more common trauma-related causes for attendance at the AED. The relatively large head makes the child top heavy and so predisposes him or her to injury.

While most head injuries are benign, a small number develop complications. The aim of management, therefore, is to identify children at risk of developing problems.

The concept of **primary** and **secondary** insult in head injury is important. Primary injury originates at the time of impact, when forces are transmitted through the brain, and is caused by rotational force, shearing force or vibrational force. Contre-coup lesions are often found diametrically opposite the point of contact. The extent to which they are present is directly related to the original force applied.

It must be remembered that these forces can be transmitted during the course of facial trauma and by forceful shaking of the child (as in non-accidental injury).

Injury sustained at this stage is usually irreversible but may be aggravated by secondary factors, many of which are controllable and preventable.

Causes of secondary brain injury include:
- Hypoxia.
- Hypovolemia.
- Cerebral edema.
- Intracranial bleeding.
- Infection.

These secondary factors often coexist and mutually predispose to further insult (**Figure 4.16**).

Good initial assessment of the head injured victim will identify those at risk of further injury or insult. It will also allow those children with low or negligible chance of further insult to avoid unnecessary investigation or admission.

The most reliable factors in determining the risk of intracranial lesions are:
- Mechanism of injury.
- Loss of consciousness.
- Skull fracture.

Determining these in children can be difficult. Certainly adequate history and examination, together with judicious use of radiology, will help. However, often no history is forthcoming and determining loss of consciousness is difficult in young children. Three questions have to be answered for every child presenting with head injury:
1. Does the child need an X-ray?
2. Does the child need admission?
3. Does the child need referral to a neurosurgeon?

In the UK, CT scanning for head injury is not performed as often as elsewhere. Usually, the child will have X-rays prior to being sent for a scan; the skull X-ray being used as a triage tool (**Figure 4.17**).

Some indications for X-ray are imprecise and are open to a degree of clinical judgement. How big for instance is a 'large laceration'? The issue of loss of consciousness in

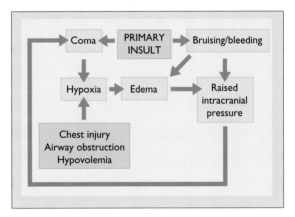

Figure 4.16
Interrelationship of factors involved in head injury

Indication for skull X-ray

1. Loss of consciousness
2. Large laceration/wound
3. Scalp hematoma
4. Clinical fracture
5. Focal signs/seizures
6. Altered level of consciousness
7. Suspected non accidental injury
8. Difficult assessment
9. Mechanism of Injury e.g. hit with hammer, fall > 5 metres

Figure 4.17

infants is addressed below, but do all parents, even if they have witnessed a blow to the head, know what loss of consciousness means? Do all medical staff know what loss of consciousness means?

Certainly, altered consciousness is important. It is especially important in the intoxicated or poisoned child where it is tempting to say that the intoxicating substance is to blame. **No allowance should be made for the intoxicant. These children should be treated as if they are comatose due to a head injury and treated as such.** However, these children can be difficult to X-ray. They may be confused and irritable. Persevering with X-rays can be fruitless. A decision will have to be made as to whether these children should be anesthetized and ventilated and then sent for a CT scan, or whether they should be admitted for observation. This decision is best made in conjunction with a neurosurgeon and will depend on local conditions and facilities.

Difficulties arise in small children in whom it can be difficult to make a full assessment. In these situations, clinical skill and expertise is vital. In particular, an estimation of whether the child has been concussed is essential. The following points suggest that an infant has been concussed:

- Failure to cry immediately.
- Going pale/limp.
- Apnea.

ADMISSION

Minor head injury accounts for a substantial number of admissions in the UK. The indications for admission are given in **Figure 4.18**; vomiting and headache are not absolute indications to admit a child while all of those in the table are. Many children vomit once or twice after sustaining a head injury but there is no cause for concern unless it becomes persistant. The vomiting may be severe enough to warrant I.V. rehydration. While few will have significant (i.e. requiring surgical treatment) intracranial causes for the vomiting, a CT scan will help exclude such lesions.

REFERRAL TO A NEUROSURGEON

In Britain, the indications to refer to a neurosurgeon really relate to the need for CT of the head (**Figure 4.19**). As mentioned earlier, better access to a CT scanner may mean that the criteria for radiography become the criteria for a CT scan. As stated above, unconscious children in whom head injury is a possibility should be discussed with a neurosurgeon.

LEVEL OF CONSCIOUSNESS

Various means exist for the assessment of level of consciousness in children:

- Glasgow Coma Scale (**Figure 4.20**)
- Glasgow Pediatric Coma Scale (**Figure 4.21**)
- AVPU (*see* **Figure 1.56**)

Indication for referral to a neurosurgeon

1. Persisting alteration in level of consciousness
2. Deteriorating level of consciousness
3. Skull fractures
4. Open fractures
5. Focal signs/seizures

Figure 4.19

Indication for admission

1. Skull fractures
2. Altered level of consciousness
3. Decreasing level of consciousness
4. Focal signs/seizures
5. Suspected non accidental injury
6. Social

Figure 4.18

Glasgow Coma Score

Value	Eye opening
4	Spontaneous
3	To voice
2	To pain
1	None
	Best motor response
6	Normal
5	Localizes to pain
4	Flexes to pain
3	Abnormal flexion
2	Extends to pain
1	None
	Best verbal response
5	Normal
4	Confused
3	Inappropriate words
2	Grunts/sounds
1	None

Figure 4.20

Figure 4.21

Glasgow Pediatric Coma Score			
Value	**Eye opening**		
	Age 0–12 months	Age >12 months	
4	Spontaneous	Spontaneous	
3	To shout	To voice	
2	To pain	To pain	
1	None	None	
	Best motor response		
	Age 0–12 months	Age >12 months	
6	Normal movements	Normal movements	
5	Localizes pain	Localizes pain	
4	Flexes to pain	Flexes to pain	
3	Abnormal flexion	Abnormal flexion	
2	Extends to pain	Extends to pain	
1	None	None	
	Best verbal response		
	Age 0–23 months	Age 24–60 months	Age >60 months
5	Smiles/cries normally	Normal	Normal
4	Cries	Inappropriate words	Disorientated
3	Inappropriate Crying	Inappropriate crying	Inappropriate words
2	Grunts	Grunts	Incomprehensible sounds
1	None	None	None

It is often impractical to use the Glasgow Coma Scale or its pediatric version in the acute phase. Here the 'AVPU' scale (**Figure 1.56**) is better and more rapid for assessing priorities. A formal assessment can be made as soon as the 'ABC of resuscitation' is under way.

MECHANISM OF INJURY

Mechanism of injury (*see* **Figure 4.17**) is also important. Single-site impacts, such as from a golf club, may be associated with depressed skull fractures. Penetrating wounds should also be taken seriously, even if the external wound is small, for example history of a dart hitting the head. The authors are aware of a case where an intranasal foreign body penetrated the cribriform plate and dura mater with subsequent meningitis. Falls from a height greater than 5m should also be taken seriously even if no obvious damage is apparent initially.

SKULL FRACTURES

As detailed above, skull fractures are associated with intracranial complications. These include hematoma formation, infection, and leptomeningeal cyst formation.

In addition, the force required to fracture the skull is considerable; the associated primary forces are therefore potentially greater leading to a greater chance of edema,

and subsequent rise in intracranial pressure.

Skull fractures (which are illustrated overleaf) can be classified as follows:

- Vault:
  —linear.
  —depressed.
  —wide/growing.
- Base

Vault fractures are usually visible on plain X-rays. Inexperienced staff can often confuse fractures with sutures and vice versa (**Figure 1.11** and **4.22**).

Depressed fractures are easy to miss and may need tangential views to confirm. CT will identify the extent of the fracture (**Figure 4.23**).

'Wide' or growing fractures are rare and suggest a fair degree of force. They may be associated with non-accidental injury (**Figure 4.24**). Wide fractures are greater than 3 mm in width on presentation. Meningeal tissue can become trapped with subsequent development of a leptomeningeal cyst.

Fractures to the base of the skull should be suspected if blood or CSF is discharged from either the nose or ears of a child. Bruising around the eyes ('racoon' or 'panda' eyes) or behind the ears ('Battles signs') should alert the

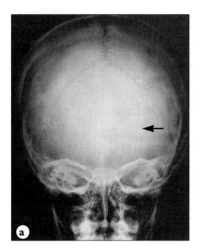

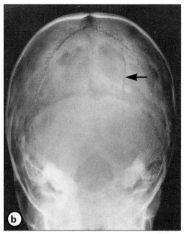

Figure 4.22 a and b
(a) Posteroanterior and (b) Towne's view of the skull showing a vertical fracture in the left occipital bone (arrows). The Towne's view confirms the site of the fracture to be in the occiput rather than the frontal bone as it clearly extends to the lambdoid suture.

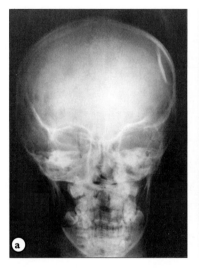

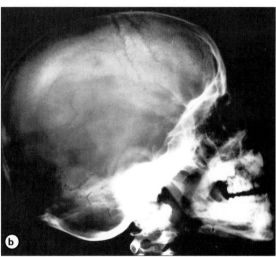

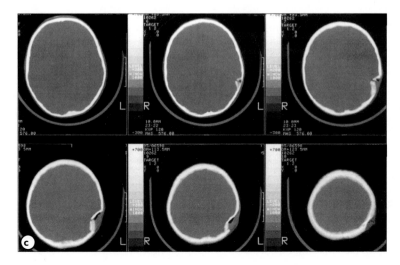

Figure 4.23 a, b and c (a) Postero-anterior and lateral (b) views of the skull showing a depressed fracture in the left parietal bone. The film (a) shows the typical sclerotic tangential appearance of the depressed fracture. View (b) shows a Mercedes Benz sign. The features are typically the result of a local impact from a sharp object. Depressed skull fracture (c) of the parietal bone. This is best evaluated with computerized tomography (CT) scanning. Note depressed-fracture fragments and air in the soft tissues peripheral to the fracture.

clinician to fractures in the base of the skull (**Figure 4.25**).

Depressed skull fractures should be discussed with a neurosurgeon following which a decision can be made as to the surgery required and its timing.

Fractures of the base of the skull are regarded as open fractures, being in communication with the ear, nose, pharynx, or mastoid air cells. Meningitis is rare but will occasionally follow such fractures; typically, pneumococci are responsible. Repeated pneumococcal meningitis with a history of head injury should lead one to suspect persistent CSF leakage.

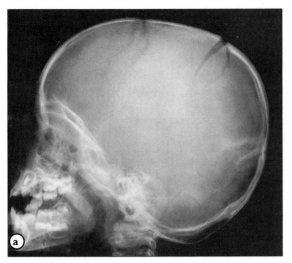 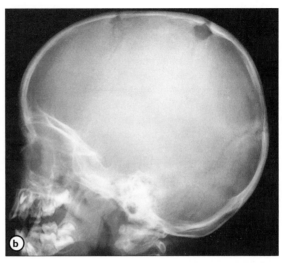

Figure 4.24 a and b
Lateral views of the skull of a child suffering from head trauma. Film (a) shows a recent fracture of the parietal bones. The fracture extends across the midline. Film (b)—taken 5 months later— shows healing of the fracture but a residual lytic area in the region of the fracture. A pulsatile swelling was present at this point and the appearances are compatible with a leptomeningeal cyst or 'growing fracture' of the skull vault.

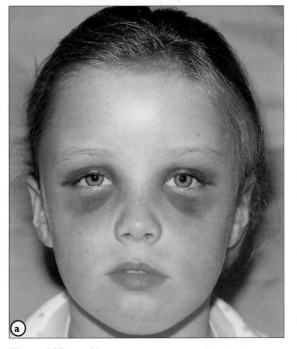 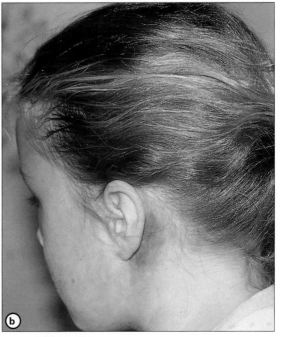

Figure 4.25 a and b
(a) This child has a suspected base-of-skull fracture. Peri-orbital bruising on both sides ('racoon' or 'panda' eyes) is associated with this type of fracture. (b) Battles signs. Bruising over the mastoid area is associated with a fracture of the base of the skull.

Vault fractures are not susceptible to infection unless associated with overlying wounds. If wounds do overlie a fracture, meticulous wound debridement is indicated.

Antibiotics may be indicated for open fractures of the skull. Local policies will dictate usage and type of drug. Typically, antibiotics will not be needed unless the dura is torn.

It is important to recognize the potential for infection to develop as meningitis will lead to increased intracranial pressure with concomitant complications.

INTRACRANIAL HEMATOMAS

Intracranial hematomas are classified as follows: extra(epi)dural, subdural, subarachnoid and intracerebral. Intracranial hematomas are associated with a rise in intracranial pressure. This pressure is manifested by a series of signs:

- Altered level of consciousness.
- Deteriorating level of consciousness.
- Focal neurologic signs.
- Pupillary changes (**Figure 4.26**)
- A lowering of the pulse and an increase in blood pressure

The extent to which these signs are present depends on the size of the lesion and the rate at which it is expanding.

EXTRADURAL HEMATOMA

Usually this is associated with a tear in the middle meningeal artery. Unfortunately, this can occur in children without concomitant fracture in the overlying bone as is often the case in adults (**Figure 4.27**).

The continued bleeding from a ruptured meningeal artery causes a rapid build up of pressure within the skull. Typically, this will initially be associated with a decrease in the level of consciousness. Often this is associated with confusion. As this persists, eye signs gradually begin to appear. Typical changes in pulse and blood pressure appear late, as do fixed, dilated pupils.

To wait for eye signs or changes in pulse or blood pressure would be too late. Any child with a decreasing level of consciousness should be discussed as a matter of urgency with neurosurgeons who can arrange further management and investigation of the child.

SUBDURAL HEMATOMA (Figure 4.28)

This may be either acute or chronic. It results from damage to the venous sinuses and is therefore associated with much less rapid bleeding than extradural hematomas.

Acute subdural hematomas are associated with considerable force, the shearing and rotational forces being large enough to tear the venous sinuses. They are also associated with intracerebral hematomas.

Chronic or subacute hematomas are associated with less severe trauma, often in the context of a bleeding diathesis, for example, hemophilia or leukemia.

INTRACEREBRAL HEMATOMA (Figure 4.29)

Intracerebral bleeding is associated with considerable force. The main effects are those of increased pressure and edema.

RAISED INTRACRANIAL PRESSURE

Following head inbjury this is due either to haematoma formation (see above), oedema or both. Oedema is due to a complicated inflammatory response which is aggravated by hypoxia, hypovolemia and infection. Of note in this context is the 'Shaken-baby syndrome'.

SHAKEN BABY SYNDROME

Small children who are shaken violently may develop numerous small areas of bruising (petechial hemorrhage) which develop into a marked edematous response. The ensuing

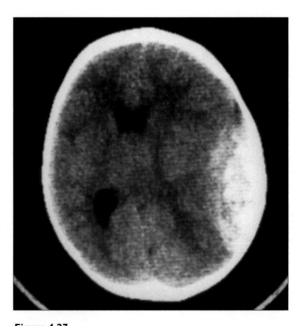

Figure 4.27
Axial computerized tomography (CT) scan of the brain in a child with an extradural hematoma. Note the high attenuating hemorrhagic collection in the right parietal epidural area. The ventricles and falx cerebri are deviated to the right.

Sequence of eye signs from a rapidly expanding intracranial lesion	
Contralateral pupil	**Ipsilateral pupil**
Normal	Constriction (seldom seen)
Normal	Dilation/sluggish response
Dilation/sluggish response	Fixed, dilated
Fixed, dilated	Fixed, dilated

Figure 4.26

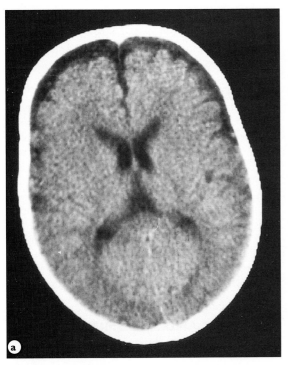

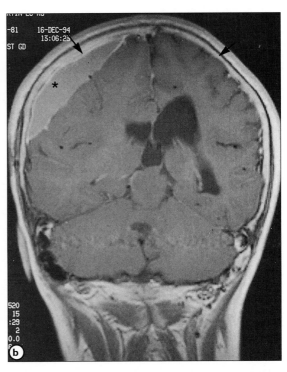

Figure 4.28 a and b

(a) Axial computerized tomography (CT) scan of the brain, in a child who had suffered a non-accidental injury, showing bilateral low density fluid overlying the frontal lobes. The appearances are indicative of subdural hematoma formation.

(b) Coronal, T1-weighted magnetic resonance imaging (MRI) scan demonstrating bilateral subdural fluid collections (arrows), but larger on the right. There is a mass effect with displacement of the midline and right lateral ventricle towards the left. The scan also shows subarachnoid blood of a different signal*.

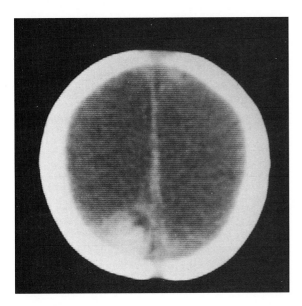

Figure 4.29

Axial computerized tomography (CT) scan of the brain of a child who had suffered a non-accidental injury. High attenuation material is seen in the falx cerebri and a more localized mass effect in the right occipital and left frontal lobes. The appearances are compatible with cerebral hematomas and subarachnoid blood.

cerebral edema is difficult to control and commonly has a poor outcome. Retinal hemorrhage often accompanies this injury (*see* Non-accidental injury).

Cerebral edema can be malignant and resistant to treatment, and is often the cause of delayed trauma deaths.

The management of post-traumatic meningitis and hydrocephalus is beyond the scope of this book.

NON-SURGICAL TREATMENT OF RAISED INTRACRANIAL PRESSURE

A hematoma may require surgical treatment. While waiting for this, several non-surgical treatments are available to buy time. These include:

- Hyperventilation
- Osmotic agents:
  Mannitol.
  Frusemide.
- Metabolism-reducing agents:
  Barbiturates.
  Hypothermia.

Their use should be discussed with a neurosurgeon before commencement. Throughout, it is important to maintain cerebral oxygenation and perfusion as best as possible.

APPROACH TO MINOR/MODERATE HEAD INJURY

The vast majority of children will attend the AED having sustained a head injury and will have recovered substantially. Symptoms such as headache, nausea, vomiting, dizziness, lethargy, and malaise are all common. In themselves they are of no significance as long as there is a full level of consciousness.

If the child has lost consciousness, or meets any of the previously described criteria, a skull X-ray should be taken. If this is normal and the child is otherwise well then he or she may be allowed home as long as home conditions permit. Head injury instructions should be given which detail symptoms and signs that might alert the parents or guardians to the development of intracranial problems. The parents should be advised to return should there be any cause for concern. Should they return the child should be fully re-examined together with reference being made to previous X-rays. If there is any concern, either on initial or subsequent visits, it may well be prudent to observe the child in an observation area for a few hours, if only to allay parental anxiety. CT may be of use in these situations.

APPROACH TO MANAGEMENT OF MAJOR HEAD INJURY

A child who is suspected of having major head injury should be admitted to the resuscitation room and the approach detailed earlier followed. Airway, breathing and circulation should be stabilized by whatever means are suitable. All other life-threatening injuries should be identified and their treatment initiated immediately. If hemorrhage is present, every effort should be made to control it by whatever means possible. Almost invariably hemorrhage will need to be stabilized before CT or neurological intervention. Certainly no child should be sent to the scan room if he or she is unstable.

Once the airway, breathing and circulation are stable and under control, it is possible to transfer the child for neurosurgical opinion, assessment and treatment.

Throughout this process orthopedic injuries, unless limb threatening, take a lower priority than injuries to the head, abdomen, or chest.

POSTCONCUSSION SYNDROME

Children who have had significant head injury will develop varying degrees of brain damage and physical impairment. Most of these children have good access to various rehabilitation services.

Of more concern is a child with mild to moderate head injury that does not require neurosurgical intervention. Often these children are admitted to pediatric or surgical wards for overnight observation and are deemed fit for discharge without any operative treatment or further intervention. Approximately 7–8% of these children will develop symptoms that interfere with their development both emotionally and educationally. These symptoms should be taken seriously with possible referral to a child psychologist. Symptoms and signs of postconcussion syndrome include headache, lethargy, poor concentration and behavioral problems.

PREVENTION

Head injury is the single leading cause of mortality in childhood following trauma. A substantial proportion of these deaths occur on the road. Children are particularly vulnerable in pedestrian/vehicle, bicycle/vehicle and vehicle/vehicle collisions. Greater use of cycle helmets and seat restraints will significantly reduce the incidence of childhood head injury. Pedestrian/vehicle injuries will be helped by education programs and by attention being focused on engineering and environmental design.

Falls from a height are another cause of head injury in childhood. Of particular concern are falls from windows and roofs of buildings. Again, education and engineering design are probably the best ways to address these issues.

THORACIC AND ABDOMINAL TRAUMA

Thoracic and abdominal trauma is relatively rare in childhood accounting for only 5% of all moderate or severe injury. In Britain, abdominal trauma is much more common than thoracic injury. Despite this, either or both can account for significant morbidity and/or mortality. In most parts of the world blunt trauma is more common than penetrating trauma.

THORACIC TRAUMA

The relatively flexible nature of the pediatric chest makes injury to the chest relatively rare. Damage to the underlying parenchymal tissues, however, can lurk behind this apparently benign facade.

Three broad categories of chest injury exist:
1. Major.
2. Moderate.
3. Minor.

In general terms, major chest injury will need urgent resuscitation and intervention with subsequent management in an intensive care setting. It is often the cause of death in the prehospital phase. Moderate chest injury will need some intervention and monitoring, and admission for observation. Minor chest injury will usually be suitable for treatment at home with minimal treatment being necessary.

MAJOR CHEST INJURY

A number of diagnoses can be grouped under this term:
- Tension pneumothorax.
- Penetrating injury.
- Major crush injury.
- Traumatic diaphragmatic hernia.

Tension pneumothorax

Tension pneumothorax is a critical emergency and is potentially life-threatening. As the pneumothorax expands it decreases the area of the lung available for gas exchange and oxygenation. Similarly, it interferes with venous return and cardiac output. The management of tension pneumothorax is considered in Chapter 1.

Penetrating injury

In Britain, penetrating chest injury is the exception rather than the rule. No matter how well the child appears on first presentation these injuries should always be triaged to a high category (*see* Chapter 1). The potential for hidden injury is vast, and sudden collapse is often catastrophic, especially if it occurs outside the resuscitation area. It should be borne in mind that the knife, missile or other sharp object can go anywhere and be deflected by ribs in unexpected directions. **What you see is not what you've got (Figure 4.30)**.

If unstable management should involve standard resuscitation procedures; the 'ABC' of resuscitation should be carried out rigorously, as previously described. Injuries potentially present will include pneumothorax (tension or otherwise), cardiac penetration with or without tamponade, major vessel damage and diaphragm injury. If the diaphragm is damaged, intra-abdominal injury is possible.

Urgent cardiothoracic opinion is indicated if any of these injuries is present or suspected. CT scanning, angiography and thoracotomy will be necessary. How, where and when these are conducted is beyond the scope of this book.

If the child is stable, appropriate imaging to detect potential vascular, cardiac or lung damage should be organized. The possibility of occult injury gradually worsening should be considered at all times. Consequently, full resuscitation equipment should always be available.

Major crush injury

Crush injury typically occurs when children are run over by a motor vehicle or heavy objects fall on top of them (**Figure 4.31**). The extent of the injury will be

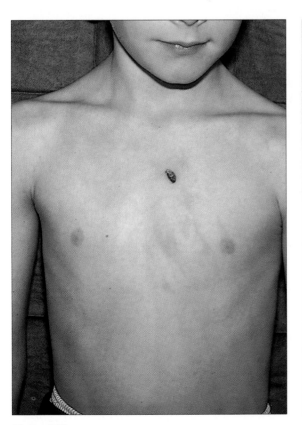

Figure 4.30
This child has sustained a penetrating injury to the anterior portion of his chest. While he looks well, and there is no obvious acute injury, the possibility of mediastinal injury and injury to the great vessels as they leave the mediastinum would have to be considered.

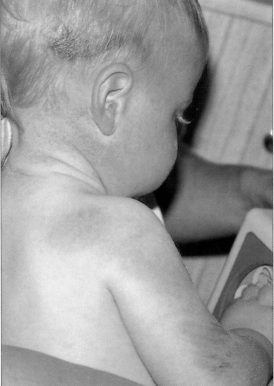

Figure 4.31
This young child has been run over by the front and rear wheels of a vehicle. He ran out of the front door as his father was reversing down the drive and was knocked over. Abrasions are visible to the arm and head. Note the petechial hemorrhage and the suffusion in the face. This child was physically well 3 hours later without any sign of intracranial or intrathoracic damage!

determined by the concomitant injuries, the duration of the insult and the forces applied.

Often the only visible external evidence that injury has occurred will be petechial hemorrhage to the neck and face (**Figure 4.32**). Lung or other injury may take time to develop fully. In addition, muscle damage may lead to myoglobinuria which, if not recognized, will lead to renal insufficiency.

All children with crush injury should be admitted until such time as all complications have been ruled out.

Traumatic diaphragmatic Hernia

This is a rare condition which can present early or late. Severe respiratory distress is usually present. Chest X-rays can be deceptive and can be confused with tension pneumothorax. If diagnosed decompression with a nasogastric tube should be attempted pending surgical treatment.

MODERATE CHEST INJURY

Moderate injury to the chest is more common than major chest injury. The injuries to be considered include:

- Simple pneumothorax.
- Lung contusion.
- Small hemothorax.
- Three or more rib fractures.
- Myocardial contusion.

Simple pneumothorax

Pneumothorax is often difficult to detect clinically. Plain chest X-ray may show a small pneumothorax often undetectable on clinical examination. Many need no active treatment but do require close observation .

Larger pneumothoraces should be drained either by aspiration or by formal chest drainage (**Figure 4.33** also *see* Chapter 1). If aspiration or observation is chosen, care

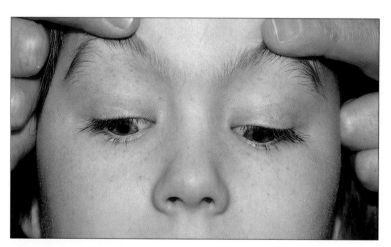

Figure 4.32
This child suffered compression forces to the chest when a door was dropped on her. The only injuries visible are bilateral petechial hemorrhages around the eyes, indicating that quite severe compressive forces were exerted on her thoracic and abdominal cavity.

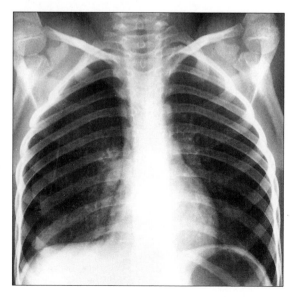

Figure 4.33
Chest X-ray in a child following a road traffic accident. A right-sided pneumothorax is present (arrowheads). Ill-defined areas of consolidation seen in the right lower lobe are compatible with pulmonary contusions.

must be taken to closely observe the child for evidence of respiratory distress. **If the child has been treated conservatively, but positive pressure ventilation is considered for any reason, consideration should be given to inserting a chest drain. This will help avoid developing a tension pneumothorax during the ventilatory process.**

Lung contusion (Figure 4.34)

Lung contusion results from any blunt chest injury. Low or falling oxygen saturations may be the first clue that the underlying injury is a contusion. Initially, supplemental oxygen may be all that is required but oxygen deficit may lead to the need for intubation and artificial ventilation.

Great care must be taken to exclude any underlying diaphragmatic rupture if lung contusions are present at the base of either lung.

Early physiotherapy should be initiated as soon as pain permits, even if this is restricted to breathing exercises.

Small hemothorax (Figure 4.35)

As with other less severe chest injuries, hemothorax may only be detected on chest radiography. Small volumes of blood may be aspirated or left to absorb. However, infec-

tion with subsequent empyema may supervene and a thoracic surgeon should be contacted early.

Three or more rib fractuers

This number of rib fractures is quite painful. There will usually be a small degree of contusion present with or without hemo/pneumothorax. These children may need to be admitted for analgesia and observation.

Children with three or more fractures have suffered quite a forceful collision to suffer this injury so other thoracic lesions should be sought and considered during the hospital stay–in particular diaphragmatic hernia.

It should be possible to administer analgesia via intercostal blocks. Repeated blocks, however, may not be well tolerated by some children so other forms of analgesia may be required. As with contusion injury, physiotherapy should be started early.

If the child needs artificial ventilation for any reason, prophylactic chest drainage should be considered. Any increase in ventilation pressure should alert the clinician to the potential for pneumothorax.

Myocardial contusion

Blunt injury to the chest, particularly if localized, may lead to myocardial contusion. Changes on electrocardiography may be the only clue. If suspected, echocar-

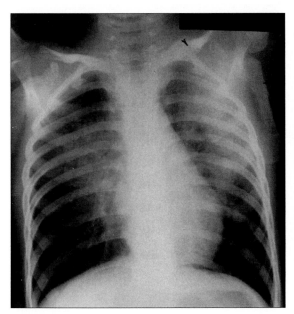

Figure 4.34
Blunt chest trauma following a road traffic accident. There is dense opacification in both lung fields due to pulmonary contusion and hemorrhage. Note fracture of the left clavicle and scapula (arrows).

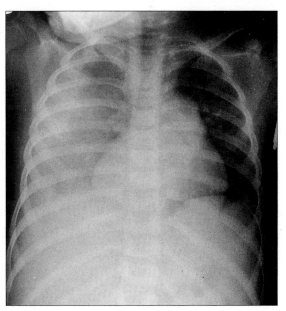

Figure 4.35
Posteroanterior chest X-ray following blunt chest trauma. This is a supine emergency film. The opaque right hemithorax represents fluid lying posteriorly in the pleural cavity. A fracture of the right 4th rib is noted. An area of consolidation is seen in the left paravertebral region. The appearances represent hemothorax following rib fracture.

diography may help detect areas of poor muscle movement. The roles of cardiac enzymes and isotope scanning are controversial.

Transient arrhythmias may be present but few are clinically relevant. The child should be admitted for observation if there is cause for concern.

MINOR CHEST INJURY

Minor chest injury is common particularly as more children are travelling restrained in seat belts with 3-point fixation (**Figure 4.36**). Injuries include: surgical emphysema, chest wall bruising and isolated rib fractures.

Surgical emphysema in the absence of pneumothorax or other injury will need little more than close observation. **If positive pressure ventilation is contemplated one should watch for pneumothorax.** Otherwise, minor chest injury will need little more than symptomatic treatment with analgesia and advice.

APPROACH TO MANAGEMENT OF CHEST INJURY

Chest injury will have been considered either as part of the primary or secondary survey, as detailed previously and resuscitation should follow the principles outlined in Chapter 1. In all major and moderate cases of chest injury, supplemental oxygen is necessary and arterial blood gases should be obtained as soon as the clinical condition permits. Treatment should not be delayed for blood gases to be analyzed although they will help future management decisions.

When transporting children with chest drains *in situ* great care must be taken not to raise the chest drain above the level of the chest. During transport situations, consideration should be given to flutter valves that do not rely on underwater seals.

ABDOMINAL TRAUMA (Figure 4.37)

Blunt trauma is the rule in Britain, with penetrating trauma occurring rarely. Other parts of the world may be less fortunate. Young children are more prone to solid organ injury due to the liver and spleen lying lower in the abdominal cavity and the rib cage providing less protection.

Blunt injury is usually caused by a direct blow to the abdomen. The extent of the injury and the organs involved will depend on the site of the blow and the force applied. Common injuries include:
- Splenic contusion/rupture.
- Hepatic contusion/rupture.
- Renal contusion/rupture.
- Bowel contusion/perforation.
- Pancreatic injury.
- Vascular injury.
- Diaphragmatic tear.
- Abdominal wall bruising.

Solid organ injury will result in hemorrhage to varying degrees. Pancreatic injury and bowel perforation will result

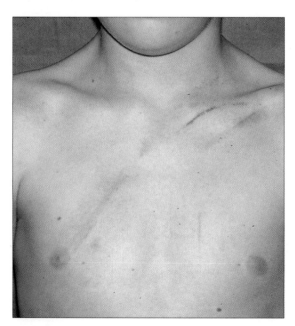

Figure 4.36
This young man has been the victim of a road traffic accident. He was a passenger in the front seat of a car travelling at 50 miles per hour. He was restrained with a seat belt (3-point fixation). The deceleration forces in the collision have thrown him forward and he has been forcibly restrained by the seat belt. These injuries indicate that a reasonably high speed collision was involved.

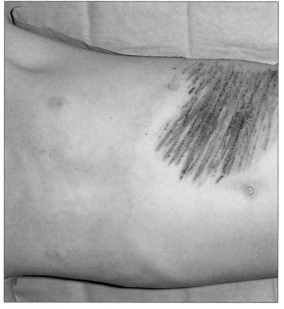

Figure 4.37
This child has been run over by a tractor trailer. He has extensive abrasions over the left upper quadrant. Clinically, renal damage, splenic damage and, possibly, bowel damage would be suspected with this injury.

in peritonitis, signs of which can take several hours to develop.

Renal injury can be detected by the presence of hematuria. Microscopic hematuria is common after all types of trauma. Frank macroscopic hematuria is less common but is indicative of a more major injury (**Figure 4.38**).

Care should be taken with the child who is unable to pass urine as bladder rupture or urethral injury may be present. While the latter injury may be diagnosed by the presence of blood at the urinary meatus, bladder rupture is difficult to identify. Often, clots from proximal damage lodge in the bladder and cause difficulty in voiding.

Examination of the child with abdominal injury can only be adequately achieved when the stomach is empty. This may require gastric decompression via a gastric tube.

It is important to examine the perineum for bruising. Urethral injuries may be sustained if the child falls astride a narrow object like a crossbar on a bicycle (**Figure 4.39**).

Symptoms and signs of intra-abdominal trauma are difficult to elicit. Pain, tenderness and bowel sounds are subjective indicators but careful and repeated examination by senior staff can help.

The modern imaging techniques of ultrasound scanning and CT have an important role to play in the diagnosis of abdominal injury. Ultrasound examination, often by repeated examination, is easy and safe but should be performed by trained personnel. Contrast studies such as intravenous urography may also be indicated if the child is stable (**Figures 4.40**). CT is, however considered the gold standard, particularly in multiple trauma, bowel rupture and pancreatic injuries.

The approach to the management of abdominal trauma will depend on the severity of the injury and the

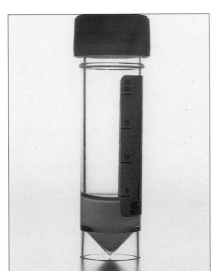

Figure 4.38
Frank hematuria following renal trauma. Further investigation of the renal tract is mandatory and other abdominal viscera (see **Figure 4.40**).

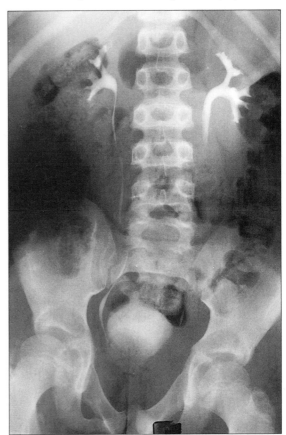

Figure 4.40
A 15-minute intravenous urography film of a child who suffered pelvic and abdominal trauma in a road traffic accident. The X-rays reveal a fracture of the right superior and inferior pubic rami and widened sacro-iliac joint. There is displacement of the bladder to the right and thickening of soft tissues in the left side of the pelvis, indicating a pelvic hematoma.

Figure 4.39
Straddle injury. This young man has landed heavily on the crossbar of his bike sustaining bruising to his perineum and scrotum. Care must be taken to exclude urethral injury, particularly if he is unable to pass urine. The temptation to pass a catheter should be resisted until a pediatric urologist has been consulted.

general condition of the child (**Figure 4.41**). Before embarking on this, one should follow the system described in Chapter 1 and earlier in this chapter, with careful attention to the 'ABC' of resuscitation. Spinal care is paramount, especially if high impact injuries are suspected.

SEAT BELT INJURIES

Recent legislation in the UK and elsewhere has made seat belt usage compulsory in both front and rear compartments of a vehicle if suitable restraints are present. This has increased the number of seat belt injuries while reducing the occurrence of other injuries.

Three-point fixation is better than lap belts. Lap belts are associated with significant intra-abdominal injury and spinal fracture, especially if high speed is involved (**Figure 4.42 and 4.80**).

A high index of suspicion is necessary in all of these cases.

PENETRATING ABDOMINAL TRAUMA

As mentioned before this is extremely rare in Britain. However, it does occur mostly from accidental impalement (**Figure 4.43**)

The size of the wound is immaterial. It is impossible to assess the depth or direction from looking at the wound. Consequently, every adjacent intra-abdominal and intrathoracic organ should be suspected as being damaged until proven otherwise.

From this observation it should be appreciated that local inspection is of little use.

Approach to the child with penetrating abdominal injury

The child should be resuscitated along previously described guidelines. If the child is stable, radiologic investigations should be instigated. This may include ultrasound assessment and CT. The child should be admitted to a high-dependency unit. The surgical team will then

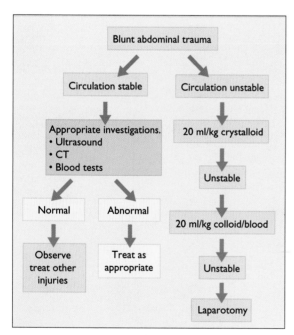

Figure 4.41
One approach to managing abdominal trauma in children.

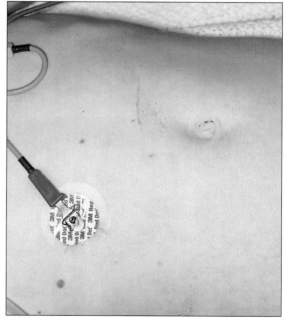

Figure 4.42
This child has extensive abdominal wall bruising sustained in a high speed collision. She was restrained by a lap seat belt.. Associated with this injury is a transverse fracture of her second lumbar vertebra associated with spinal cord damage. All children with this history and examination findings should have spinal cord injury strongly suspected and full spinal precautions instituted as described earlier (see also **Figure 4.80**).

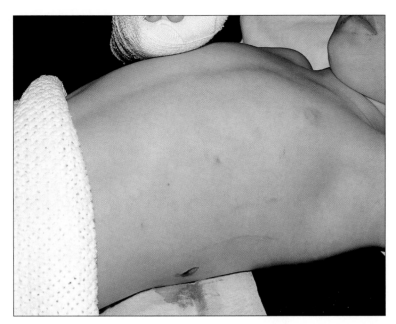

Figure 4.43
This young man has a penetrating injury to the left renal area–he was stabbed by a school friend in a row. There is no indication as to whether this wound has gone upwards into the chest, transversely into the spleen or kidney or has even gone deeply at all.

decide on further management of the wound and the treatment of any internal injury.

If the child is shocked or unstable urgent laparotomy is indicated and all injuries should be dealt with as appropriate.

PEDIATRIC FRACTURE CARE

PEDIATRIC SKELETAL SYSTEM
The pediatric skeleton differs from the adult skeleton both anatomically and physiologically. These differences have important implications for the diagnosis and treatment of pediatric fractures.

ANATOMICAL DIFFERENCES
The most striking difference between the pediatric skeleton and that of the fully mature skeleton is the presence of epiphyseal growing areas. The changes with age probably give rise to some of the most difficult dilemmas in pediatric trauma care.

With regard to the importance of therapy, the most vital factor is the need to identify and classify the various combinations of fracture in and around the epiphyses.

Fractures can and do involve the epiphyseal plate, the area distal to the epiphyseal plate, the area proximal to the epiphyseal plate or any of these in combination. Each of these injuries has different abilities to heal. The problem lies in how they heal and the degree of growth arrest which accompanies each of these injuries.

CLASSIFICATION OF FRACTURES
The most widely used classification of fractures around the epiphyseal region is the Salter–Harris classification of epiphyseal injury. This is divided into five categories: a Salter–Harris I fracture has the best prognosis and a Salter–Harris V fracture the worst prognosis (**Figure 4.44**).

Salter–Harris I fracture
The Salter–Harris I fracture is basically little more than bruising to the epiphyseal plate. It is commonly found around the wrist joint and the ankle joint (lateral malleolar area). These injuries are probably underdiagnosed. In the adult population, the mechanism of injury results in significant ligamentous injury. In children, the ligament is stronger than the epiphyseal area. The damage is due to forces applied through the area of the epiphysis rather than the ligament.

The only abnormality visible on X-ray is a degree of soft tissue swelling around the joint and the epiphyseal plate (**Figure 4.44** and **4.45**). Ultrasound examination can show lesions not visible on plain films.

Salter–Harris II fracture
Salter–Harris II fractures start in the metaphysis and continue into the epiphyseal plate (**Figure 4.44** and **4.46**). They usually heal up well, but occasionally require manipulation. They are frequently found around the ankles, wrist and base of the finger.

Salter–Harris III fracture
Salter–Harris III fractures occur in the epiphysis distal to the epiphyseal plate and extend into the joint surface. The most common area for these to occur is in the ankle joint. These fractures have a higher degree of premature fusion of the epiphyseal plate around the fracture site (**Figure 4.44** and **4.47**). Accurate reduction with internal fixation may be required.

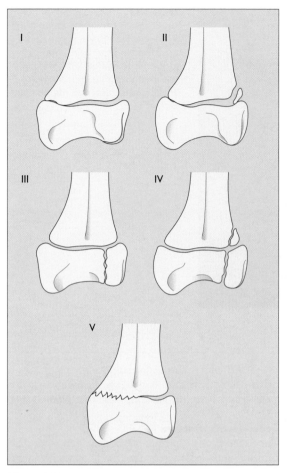

Figure 4.44
Salter–Harris classification of epiphyseal injury. See main text for further explanation.

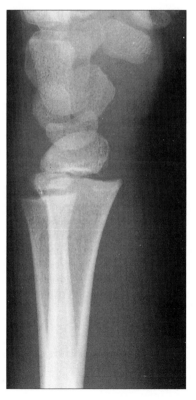

Figure 4.45
Anteroposterior view of the ankle showing widening of the epiphyseal plate–a classical Salter–Harris type I injury. An associated greenstick fracture of the distal fibula is noted.

Figure 4.46
Lateral view of the wrist. The X-ray demonstrates a Salter–Harris type II fracture with minor dorsal displacement of the distal epiphysis together with a small fracture fragment from the radial metaphysis.

Salter–Harris IV fracture

Salter–Harris IV fractures start at the joint surface and continue through the epiphyseal plate right up into the metaphysis of the bone (**Figure 4.44** and **4.48**). Again, these must be accurately reduced to reduce premature fusion and growth arrest.

Salter–Harris V fracture

Salter–Harris V fractures result in considerable damage and usually consist of crushing injuries to the epiphyseal plate area. They can be indistinguishable from Salter–Harris I injuries. They may only be noticed after growth arrest has taken place. One of the more common types of injury (which is probably not really a grade V injury at all) is a slipped upper femoral epiphysis. Other areas where the injury can be missed include the medial and lateral epicondyles, particularly when associated with dislocated elbows (**Figure 4.44**).

Epiphyseal injuries may result in premature growth fusion. Consequently, these fractures need to be followed-up with a great degree of care and by personnel with experience in their management.

PHYSIOLOGICAL DIFFERENCES

The skeleton of a child undergoes active growth and has a higher metabolic rate than in an adult bone. This leads to greater rapidity of healing and abundant callus at fracture

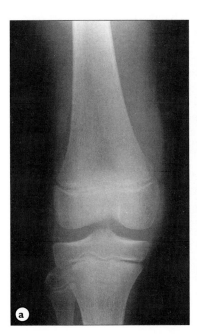

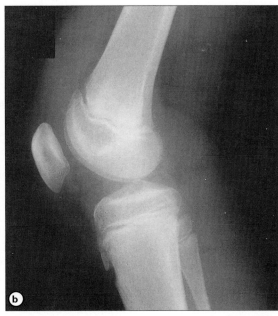

Figure 4.47 a and b Anteroposterior and lateral views of the right knee. There is a faint vertical lucent fracture involving the mid part of the distal femoral epiphysis seen on the AP film. This would be classified as a Salter–Harris Type III fracture. No fracture is seen on the lateral film (b), but there is a large suprapatellar joint effusion.

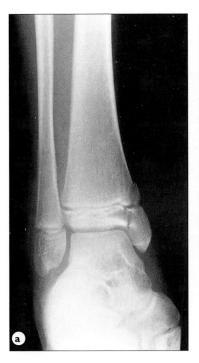

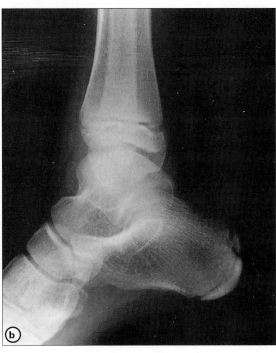

Figure 4.48 a and b Anteroposterior and lateral views of the distal tibia and fibula. The AP film clearly shows a Salter–Harris Type IV type injury of the distal tibia with a fracture extending vertically through the metaphysis and epiphysis crossing the epiphyseal line.

sites. This is aided by children having a more active periosteum than do adults. As a consequence, there is a greater chance of malunion taking place if anatomic alignment is not maintained adequately by whatever means chosen.

One of the phenomena associated with pediatric skeletal injury is the potential for bones to remodel. It should be borne in mind that remodeling is not the rule and will only occur in certain circumstances. The conditions required for bone remodeling to occur are:

- fractures close to the epiphyseal plate
- fractures in the line of motion of the joint
- more than 2 years remaining before final fusion of the epiphysis.

It should be noted that rotational deformities in fractures in the midshaft of the bone will not result in remodeling to any great extent.

OTHER TYPES OF FRACTURE

Open fracture

Open (or compound) fractures are relatively rare in childhood. The injury can be caused in one of two ways:

1. The bone is fractured from outward to inward, typically in a crush or penetrating injury (**Figure 4.49**).
2. From inward to outward where the rotation of twisting forces applied through the bone cause the bone to fracture and subsequently pierce the skin (**Figure 4.50**).

All open fractures should be managed with care as the possibility of osteomyelitis is high, especially if adequate debridement is not carried out.

Greenstick fracture

Greenstick fractures are peculiar to childhood. They are the result of forces being applied to the pediatric skeleton.

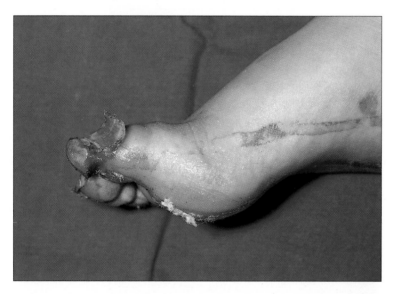

Figure 4.49
Crush injury. This great toe has been injured by a heavy weight dropping on top of it. The skin has broken and the underlying bones are fractured by external forces.

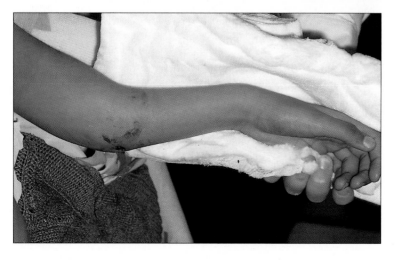

Figure 4.50
Open (compound) fracture of forearm. Bone has penetrated the skin creating a potential for infection.

The peculiar anatomic and physiologic details alluded to above result in the buckling-type deformity with minimal cortical damage. Usually these fractures are visible as just a small bulge in the periosteum and cortex (*see* **Figure 4.45**). They are easy to miss. The consequence of missing such a fracture is very minor. Usually the child will have a period of pain for a couple of weeks which gradually goes away. Some children are relatively pain-free, depending on the pain threshold of the child.

Despite this, it is our practice to immobilize these fractures in a plaster cast for a few weeks, mainly for pain relief and comfort.

PRINCIPLES OF FRACTURE CARE

Once diagnosis of a fracture has been made it is important to realize that many options for treatment are available. The doctor has to decide whether the fracture is in an acceptable position or whether it requires reduction. Many fractures do not require any form of rigid immobilization but may be treated quite adequately by sling, collar and cuff and other forms of strapping. The skill of pediatric fracture care is knowing which fracture can be treated in which manner.

Rigid casts

Casting is a skill that is difficult to acquire and once acquired requires practice to maintain. Traditionally, plaster casts are applied to immobilize the joint below and above the fracture. Variations on this in the upper limb include wrists placed in supination and pronation to help maintain the fracture in position against the counter traction of the muscles proactive at the fracture site.

Various types of casting material are now available (**Figure 4.51**). Plaster of Paris is the oldest casting material available. It is easy to use, gives rise to smooth edges and is easy to remove. Its disadvantages are that it is heavy, it must not be allowed to get wet, and is prone to breaking down.

Resin and fiberglass casts are coming much more into fashion. Apart from being available in attractive colors they are very rigid, light and not prone to disintegration (in the same way that plaster of Paris casts are). They can be difficult to handle and apply and are relatively more expensive than a plaster of Paris cast. It is up to individual departments to choose their preferred method of casting.

A small layer of wool under the cast will allow for swelling at the fracture site. It is important that the amount of wool does not prevent the plaster from being moulded against the fracture site.

Complications from plaster casts must be recognized. It should be borne in mind that any limb placed in a plaster cast, following an injury, may swell. If the swelling is allowed to persist against the rigid plaster cast, a small degree of ischemia sets in. This in turn aggravates the swelling process and a downward spiral ensues. This gives rise to severe pain in the limb under the cast.

It is important at this stage to split the plaster cast down to the skin, and over the entire length of the plaster, and to stretch the cast; this maneuver should be performed as early and as rapidly as possible (Figure 4.52).

This is much easier to do with plaster of Paris casts than resin casts. Once the plaster cast is split the child should have the limb elevated and circulation assessed in approximately half an hour. The most effective way to assess the circulation is to stretch the fingers or toes. If this aggravates the pain then the muscle compartment is under pressure and the plaster must be removed. At this stage, the child should be referred to an orthopedic surgeon who may consider monitoring pressure in the muscle compartment involved. The consequences of failing to follow this procedure are that the child is likely to develop a Volkmann's ischemic contracture.

For the reasons alluded to above, it is not adequate to treat a child in plaster with analgesia alone. The plaster must be split to allow swelling to take place and only when this has been done, and there is absolutely no evidence of compartment injury, should analgesia be given.

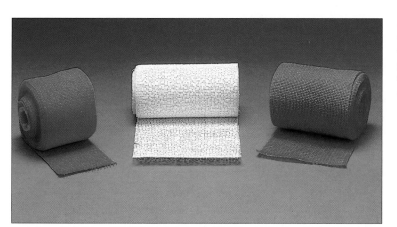

Figure 4.51

Casting materials. The central white traditional plaster of Paris is flanked by resin casts. Resin casts come in different colors which make them attractive to children.

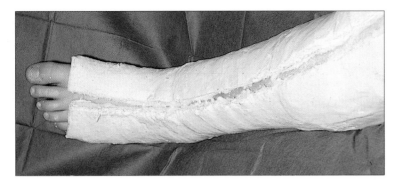

Figure 4.52
A long leg plaster cast which has been split along its entirety and the cast widened to allow for swelling to take place. If the limb still elicits pain on dorsiflexing of the toes, the cast must be removed and consideration given to compartment syndrome.

Traction splints

Fractured femurs are commonly treated in a Thomas splint in conjunction with various modifications of balanced traction. In the AED, it is sufficient to put the child in a Thomas splint with traction through the length of the leg applied using skin traction (**Figure 4.53**). Counter-traction is applied against the ischium. Sufficient tension should be applied through the strings at the end to render the limb motionless when the splint is moved.

The ring at the proximal end should be of sufficient diameter to go round the swollen femur and not to 'dig in' at any point.

Collar and cuff/slings

These are suitable for the treatment of upper limb injury. If used, it is important that the child has some other extra degree of support. This invariably means that the limb is kept below the clothes until the fracture has started to unite (**Figure 4.54**). The disadvantage of using this method is that the skin may excoriate in the axilla or in the antecubital fossa. Should this happen the child should be brought back to the AED to be assessed further.

Other methods of fracture care

Some minor fractures of the lower limb and foot may be treated with simple tubular elastic bandages and kept non-weight bearing on crutches. Once the pain begins to subside it is possible to start mobilizing the child effectively. Metatarsal fractures, calcaneal fractures and fractures of the ankle are particularly suitable for this type of treatment. It should be borne in mind that the fractures must essentially be undisplaced and there should be little chance of displacement should the child weight-bear early.

Fractures not suitable for treatment in any of these forms should be referred for more appropriate treatment.

INDIVIDUAL FRACTURES IN THE UPPER LIMB

Fractured clavicle

A fractured clavicle is one of the more common injuries of childhood. Typically, the injury results from a fall onto the shoulder. The injury can be very difficult to diagnose in small children both clinically and radiologically. Clinical examination will reveal tenderness along the shaft of the clavicle. Radiology may show a small kink in the clavicle. It may not be until a palpable callus is formed that the fracture is actually apparent (**Figures 4.55 and 4.56**).

Treatment is by simple immobilization in a sling either with or without a figure-of-eight bandage. As detailed above, the sling should be worn under the clothes for about 10 days after which the movements of the childs shoulder should gradually resume. This is a very painful injury and adequate analgesia should be prescribed. Sleeping propped up may be beneficial and give the child (and parents) a good night's sleep.

Parents often become very concerned about the callus formation in the bone which develops after 7–10 days. It is not unusual for anxious parents to be more concerned

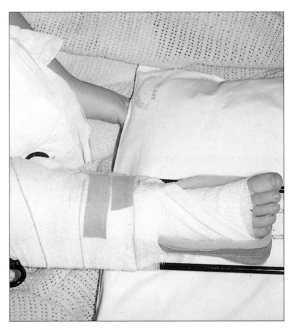

Figure 4.53
Thomas splint *in situ* prior to going to X-ray or the ward.

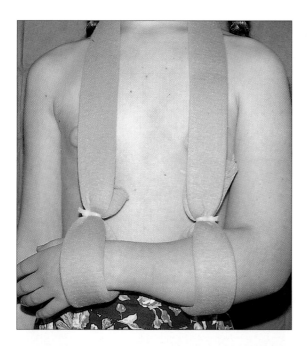

Figure 4.54
This child has a fracture around the elbow region which has been splinted in a collar and cuff. This double collar and cuff arrangement is possibly more comfortable around the neck.

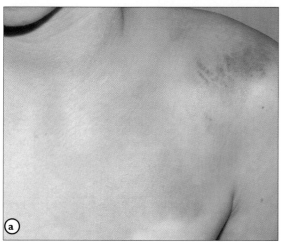

Figure 4.55 a
This young man has sustained a nasty fracture of the clavicle with extensive soft tissue swelling.

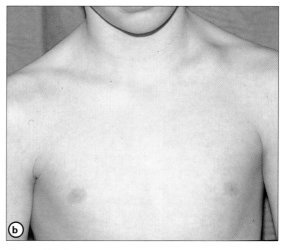

Figure 4.55 b
The same child as in Figure 4.55a. There is prominent swelling over the left clavicle where callus is forming 3 weeks later.

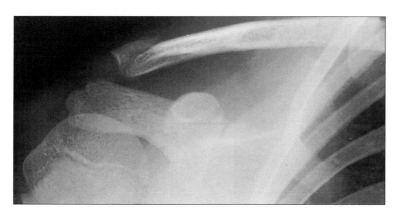

Figure 4.56
Radiograph demonstrating a fracture of the lateral third of the clavicle.

about the palpable swelling than the fall or the fracture and to bring the child back to the department. Advice about this early in treatment will allay fears.

Fracture to the neck of the humerus

These fractures range from a simple greenstick fracture to one where the shaft is almost completely separated from the head of the humerus (**Figure 4.57**). These fractures heal up remarkably well. Usually all that is required is for the arm to be supported in a collar and cuff with the wrist higher than the elbow. The sling should be worn under the clothes for several weeks with the child allowed to mobilize within the limits of pain. The first few days can be quite painful and it may be necessary to admit the child for analgesia.

Shaft of humerus

Fracture of the shaft of the humerus is occasionally associated with damage to the radial nerve. The function of this nerve should be checked as soon as possible after the injury is diagnosed. Repair of the nerve itself is seldom indicated if there is a lesion present. However, expert advice should be taken regarding this before making a final decision (**Figure 4.58**).

It is difficult to immobilize this fracture. A 'U-slab' may provide some relief. However, this plaster is difficult to apply. Again, the child may require admission for pain relief.

Fractures around the elbow

Many fractures occur around the elbow joint. The changing appearance of the elbow joint with age can make some of these fractures difficult to diagnose (**Figure 4.59**).

Supracondylar fracture

This is caused by a fall on the outstretched arm. The force continues through the arm and elbow and forces the distal end of the humerus backwards. The fracture can range from one where there is a tiny greenstick element present to almost complete separation of the distal end of the humerus from the proximal shaft. Rotatory elements complicate this latter injury.

Minor fractures may be treated in a collar and cuff (**Figure 4.54**). The more severe the injury, the more necessary it is to consider urgent reduction. Supracondylar fractures are associated with damage to the brachial artery. Pulsation of the radial artery distally must be documented as soon as the injury is suspected. Absence of a radial pulse is serious. Manipulation should be undertaken as an emergency.

Such fractures should usually be reduced where facilities for exploration of the artery also exist.

While also possible, injuries to the median, ulnar, or radial nerves seem to occur with much less frequency with this type of injury than might be expected in view of the nature of the injury.

Flexion deformity also occurs, but less often. The principles of treatment are the same.

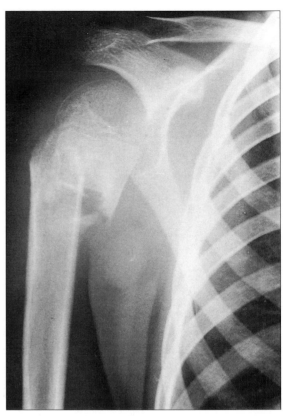

Figure 4.57
Radiograph of the right shoulder. The X-ray depicts a comminuted fracture of the surgical neck of the humerus. A lateral film, either as a transthoracic or axial view, would be indicated to demonstrate any significant displacement of the fragments.

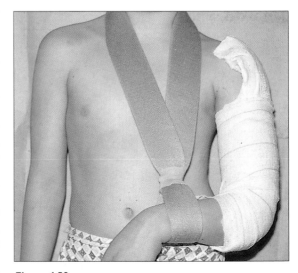

Figure 4.58
Fractured shaft of humerus with associated radial nerve palsy. The child is unable to extend his wrist or hand.

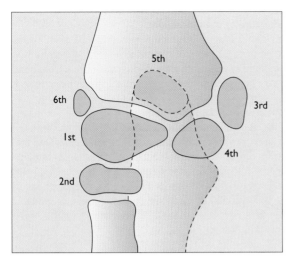

Figure 4.59
Order in which epiphyses appear around the elbow.
1st: Capitellum. 2nd Radial head. 3rd Medial epicondyle. 4th Trochlea.
5th Olecranon. 6th Lateral epicondyle.

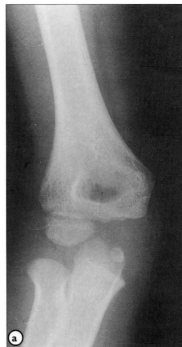

Figure 4.60 a and b
(a) Anteroposterior and (b) lateral views of the elbow. The appearances illustrate an avulsion of the medial epicondyle of the humerus which is clearly shown lying within the joint space (arrows). A metaphyseal fragment of bone is seen on the lateral image lying posterior to the distal humerus.

Avulsion of the medial epicondyle

The medial epicondyle is the more common of the two epicondyles to be injured. It is associated with dislocation of the elbow but can also occur on its own (**Figure 4.60**). The injury is often missed by inexperienced doctors. Diagnosis can be difficult but should be suspected if the gap between the medial epicondyle and the distal end of the medial border of the humerus is greater than 1 mm. Again extensive soft tissue swelling is usually present. The medial epicondyle may lie within the joint space and the X-ray should be inspected closely to detect this complication. The ulnar nerve should be examined distal to the fracture site.

Lateral epicondylar injury

This is much less common than the medial epicondylar injury. It should again be suspected if there is soft tissue injury around the elbow joint or there is any degree of instability around the joint itself.

TREATMENT

All epicondylar injuries should be referred for orthopedic opinion.

Dislocation of the elbow

Apart from dislocation of the finger, this is one of the most common dislocations which occur in childhood. It can be diagnosed clinically by the awkward shape of the elbow (**Figure 4.61**).

One may be tempted to reduce this injury in the AED. It is technically feasible to do this. However, it can be very

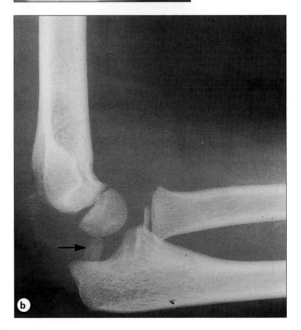

difficult to examine the elbow afterwards if the child is not under general anesthesia. Once the elbow is reduced, it is important to check stability of the joint and also the position of the medial and lateral epicondyle (**Figure 4.62**). Therefore, it is better for this injury to be reduced under anesthesia where facilities for further treatment exist.

Monteggia fracture

A Monteggia fracture is an injury of the ulna with dislocation and/or subluxation of the radial head. Many varieties exist. The radial head can be dislocated anteriorly, laterally or posteriorly. Fractures of the proximal end of the ulna and the olecranon can also be associated with minor fractures of the radial head and these must be classed again as a variant of a Monteggia fracture.

Radiologically, all elbow injuries should be scrutinized to ensure that the radial head is in alignment with the capitellum (**Figure 4.63**).

Monteggia fractures should be referred for orthopedic treatment.

Fracture of the olecranon

Fractures of the olecranon/proximal ulna are often associated with fractures of the radial head. These should be splinted in a cast with early follow-up arranged. If the ulnar fragments are separated, open reduction may be necessary.

Fractures of the radial head/neck

Impaction fractures of the radial neck are common and often extend into the epiphyseal area of the radial head. These fractures can give rise to significant loss of pronation and supination. Minor degrees of impaction may heal well. Otherwise these injuries should be discussed with an orthopeadic surgeon, who can decide on the operative treatment or not.

It is important to look for associated fractures of the proximal ulna.

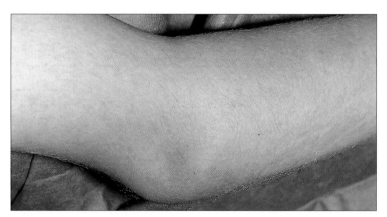

Figure 4.61
Dislocation of the elbow with typical deformity.

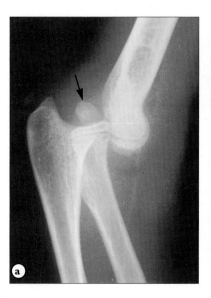 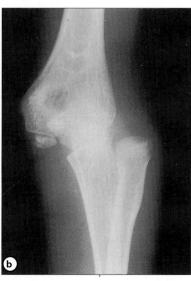

Figure 4.62 a and b
(a) lateral view of the elbow. (b) AP views of the elbow.
The X-rays demonstrate a typical posterior dislocation of the elbow. The X-rays also reveal an avulsed medical epicondyle which lies within the joint space (arrow).

Fractures of the shaft of the radius and ulna

Fractures of the shaft of the radius and ulna can be deceptive in the degree of angulation present. These injuries do not remodel well. Angled fractures should be referred for orthopedic opinion (**Figure 4.64**).

Beware the isolated fracture of the ulna. One is duty bound to exclude an associated dislocation/subluxation of the radial head (*see* above).

Galeazzi fracture

This is the reverse of the Monteggia fracture. Here there is a fracture of the shaft of the radius with subluxation of the distal end of the ulna. This is a much rarer injury. Often a Salter–Harris I fracture of the distal radius will be present with a subluxed ulna. Once diagnosed, referral should be made to the orthopedic surgeons who will consider further management.

Fractures to the distal end of the radius

These are one of the most common fractures found in childhood. Two basic types of injury are present:
1. Hyperextension (**Figure 4.65**).
2. Hyperflexion.

Hyperextension injuries are similar to those that occur in adults. The hyperflexion injuries are equivalent to a Smith's type injury which occurs in adults.

Most of these injuries can be treated in a cast. If there is pain on pronation/supination, then the child is better

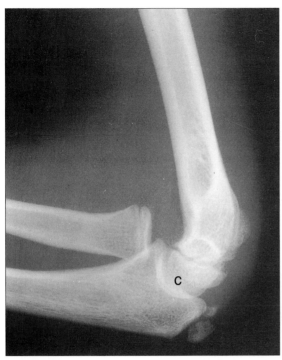

Figure 4.63
Lateral view of the elbow showing superior dislocation of the proximal radius. A line drawn along the shaft of the radius should intersect the capitellum (c). In this case, the projected line falls superior indicating a dislocation.

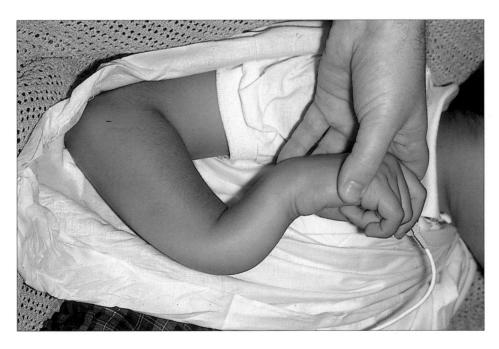

Figure 4.64
Grossly deformed midshaft fracture of the radius and ulna. This is almost impossible to splint adequately.

placed in a cast above the elbow. If the child is relatively comfortable on pronation and supination then brow–elbow cast is usually all that is required. However, once the cast is in place it is prudent to assess the child to see if there is any pain. Any increase in pain on movement of the elbow should lead one to extend the cast to above the elbow.

If there is displacement or angulation at the fracture site the child should be referred for reduction under general anaesthesia or at the very least sent for an orthopedic assessment as to whether remodeling might occur (**Figure 4.66**).

FRACTURES IN THE LOWER LIMB
Fractures of the femur
Femoral fractures are again relatively common in childhood. Typically, the shaft is fractured, with fractures of the neck and trochanteric area being relatively rare in childhood.

Fractures of the shaft of the femur
Fractures of the shaft of the femur can be either transverse, spiral or oblique. They are extremely painful and analgesia is required as a matter of urgency before any further treatment is given. This fracture is amenable to femoral nerve block which should be achieved as soon as possible (*see* Figure 4.4).

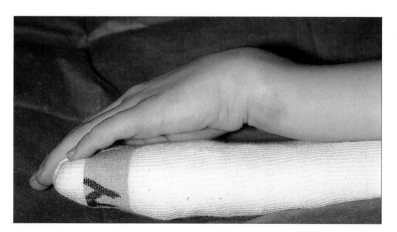

Figure 4.65
Typical hyperextension injury to the distal radius and ulna showing a mild degree of dorsal angulation.

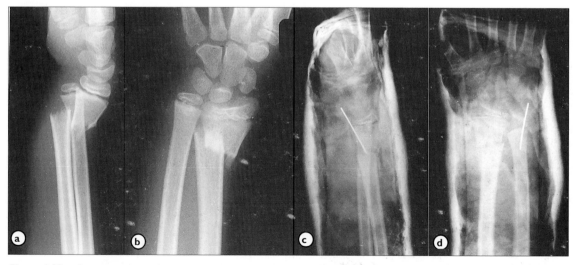

Figure 4.66 a–d
(a) Anteroposterior and (b) lateral views of the wrist. There is transverse fracture of the distal radial metaphysis with dorsal displacement of the distal fragment; (c) and (d) reveal good position of the radius and ulna in plaster following treatment.

During manipulation of the distal radius, a fracture of the distal ulna occurred. Radiographs (c) and (d) thus show the pin in position for the fixation of the second iatrogenic fracture.

Once the nerve is blocked the child should be placed in a Thomas splint and traction applied (*see* **Figure 4.6**). It is then permissible to X-ray the child. All fractures should be referred to an orthopedic surgeon for further management.

Fractures of the lower end of the femur

Fractures of the lower end of the femur are occasionally associated with vascular damage. It is important, therefore, to assess pulses distal to the femur.

In addition, Salter–Harris I fractures may occur at the distal end of the femur. These are difficult to determine and can often be confused with ligamentous injuries if adequate care in examination is not taken.

Intra-articular fractures of the knee

Two types of intra-articular fractures occur:
1. Those involving the femoral condyles (**Figures 4.47a and b, 4.67**).
2. Those involving the tibial plateau (**Figure 4.68**).

Both types of injury are associated with gross knee effusions. The knee bleeds very quickly and the joint will be very tense by the time the child presents.

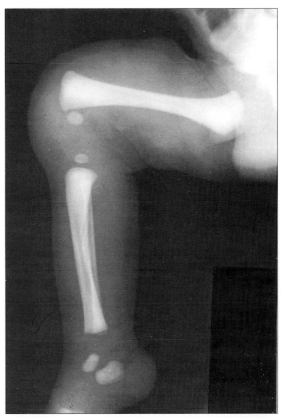

Figure 4.67
Lateral view of the knee of a new-born baby. This shows a Salter–Harris Type II injury of the distal femur with total dislocation of the distal femoral epiphysis plus metaphyseal fragment.

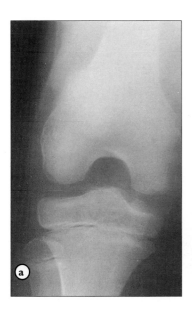

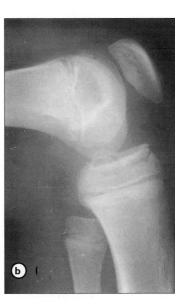

Figure 4.68 a and b
(a) Anteroposterior and (b) lateral views of the knee demonstrating a fracture of the anterior tibial plateau. A suprapatellar joint effusion is present.

Consequently, any child presenting with an acute hemarthrosis should be suspected of having one of these two injuries. Both types of fracture require specialist assessment.

Patellar fractures

Fractures of the patella are rare in childhood. Fractures can occur at either the inferior pole or transversely (**Figure 4.69 a**). Difficulty can arise in diagnosis if developmental abnormalities are present (**Figure 4.69 a**).

Simple fractures can be managed in a plaster cylinder. More complicated fractures, where there is separation, may need to be internally fixed and should be discussed with an orthopedic surgeon (**Figure 4.70 a and b**).

Dislocated patella

Dislocation of the patella is more common in girls than boys. Often the dislocation has been reduced by the time the child presents making diagnosis difficult. Skyline views of the patella are difficult to achieve but can help the diagnosis. Flakes of avulsed periosteum and bone may be visible on the medial border of the patella.

If the dislocated patella has been reduced, and the diagnosis is suspected, the child should be treated in a well-padded leg cylinder. If the patella is still dislocated it should be reduced as a matter of urgency and the above treatment given. Again, X-rays should be taken prior to any immobilization in a plaster cast.

Recurrent dislocation is common after the initial injury. Orthopedic follow-up is indicated.

Fracture to the shaft of the tibia

Tibial fractures may be spiral, oblique or transverse. They are usually quite painful and analgesia should be given as a matter of routine. The limb should be splinted in a box-

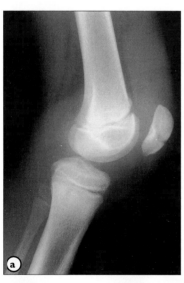

Figure 4.69 a
Lateral view of the knee. This demonstrates a transverse fracture through the midpole of the patella with an associated suprapatellar joint effusion.

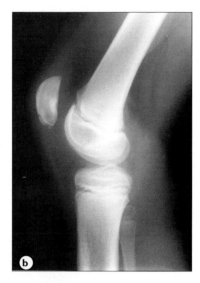

Figure 4.69 b
This view shows a normal variant, i.e. a secondary ossification center of the lower pole of the patella. There is no associated soft tissue swelling and the appearances must not be regarded as a fracture.

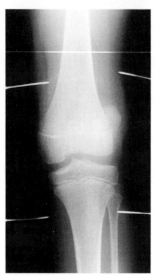
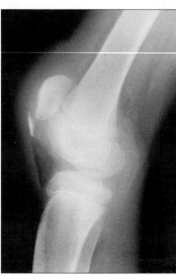

Figure 4.70
Anteroposterior and lateral views of the left knee. The X-rays illustrate a vertical fracture through the patella with separation of the two lateral fragments.

splint prior to X-ray (**Figure 4.7**). Arterial pulses should be palpated distal to the fracture and documented (**Figure 4.71**). In larger children, it can be difficult to image the knee and ankle on one film, but this should be achieved wherever possible.

Displaced fractures will usually require some degree of manipulation and consequently children should be referred to an orthopedic surgeon who will conduct the procedure under general anaesthetic.

Undisplaced fractures or fractures with a minor degree of displacement are suitable for treatment in long leg casts. These can be very difficult to apply and a general anesthetic may be required to do this adequately and humanely. Once in the cast the leg should be X-rayed to ensure that fracture alignment has been maintained. Larger children should certainly be admitted for this procedure. This will allow mobilization to be attempted on crutches over a period of time. Smaller children or children in whom the degree of swelling is minimal may be suitable for treatment at home. This will depend on local policies.

Open fractures, and those fractures associated with tissue loss, may require open reduction and fixation, either internally or externally.

Fibular fractures

The fibula is rarely fractured but, occasionally, a direct blow to the shaft can result in an angular deformity. This is usually greenstick in origin and will normally resolve with time. Often all that is needed is to protect the limb in a light cast. Reduction and straightening of the fibula may be indicated and this should be discussed with an orthopedic surgeon.

Ankle fractures

The ankle is prone to several types of injury. The most common is a Salter–Harris I fracture to the lateral malleolus. It is usually associated with a fair degree of swelling and X-ray is usually quite normal apart from soft tissue swelling (**Figure 4.72 a–c**).

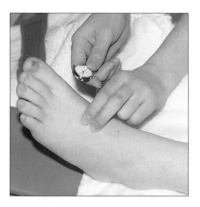

Figure 4.71
The pulse should be checked in all children with fractures of the lower limb. Here the dorsalis pedis pulse is being palpated.

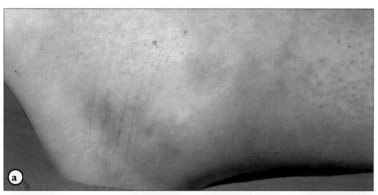

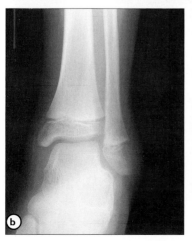

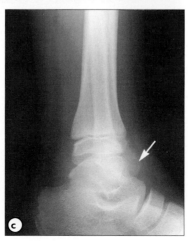

Figure 4.72 a–c
(a) Extensive soft tissue swelling associated with pitting edema. No fracture was seen on plain radiography.
(b) Anteroposterior and (c) lateral views of the ankle of a child suffering a twisting injury. The lateral film clearly demonstrates a soft tissue density teardrop lying anterior to the ankle joint (arrow). This is pathognomonic of an ankle joint effusion. There was no fracture demonstrated.

Avulsion fractures of the distal part of the fibula

Inversion injuries may result in small fragments being avulsed from the distal lateral malleolus. Most children can be managed with tubular elastic bandages and non-weight-bearing on crutches. Mobilization should be supported by a physiotherapist. Occasionally, some children will not tolerate this and a cast should be applied for pain relief. However, if a cast is applied in these circumstances it should be removed as soon as pain subsides at which point the child can be mobilized at physiotherapy. These measures will help prevent reflex sympathetic dystrophy.

OTHER FRACTURES

Medial malleolar fractures tend to be Salter–Harris III type injuries, although occasionally they are of the Salter–Harris IV type (*see* **Figure 4.48**). They should be referred to an orthopedic surgeon as a matter of course since internal fixation may be required.

Toddler's fracture of the tibia

Small children, particularly those between the ages of 1 and 3 years, are prone to this type of injury (*see* the Limping Child: Chapter 5).

Typically, the child presents without any great history of trauma but has a history of limping for 24 to 48 hours. Palpation of the tibia may reveal areas of tenderness, but often this is absent. Radiographs taken of the lower limb reveal no bony injury. The rest of the limb is also normal. If suspected the child should be brought back in 10 days when further X-rays may reveal evidence of a healing fracture (**Figure 4.73**). This is visible in the form of a periosteal reaction and

at this stage a small fracture line may be visible. Often, in retrospect, it is possible to see a hairline crack in the original film. Children with this type of injury usually come to no harm, even if no active treatment is prescribed.

Calcaneal fractures

Fracture to the calcaneum results from a fall or jump from a height on to the flat of the foot. All children with this type of injury should have a calcaneal fracture suspected. The history is not always obtained. For this reason all ankle X-rays should be scrutinized for evidence of calcaneal injury. If suspected, specific views of the calcaneum should be requested (**Figure 4.74**).

Once diagnosed, the treatment will depend on the child, the family and the degree of swelling present. If the swelling is marked and the tenderness severe, the child should be admitted for elevation and bed rest. Otherwise the child can be allowed home in a light cast and a follow-up arranged.

Minor undisplaced fractures of the calcaneum may be treated in an elastic tubular bandage and the child mobilized on crutches, non-weight-bearing on the injured leg.

The origin of calcaneal injuries is such that the child has usually jumped from a height. Children who have jumped from a significant height and landed on their heels are prone to further injury. In particular, knee, neck of femur, sacroiliac joints and spinal injuries are associated with calcaneal fractures. Children with this injury should have all of these areas examined clinically and if there is any concern they should be investigated radiologically and treated accordingly.

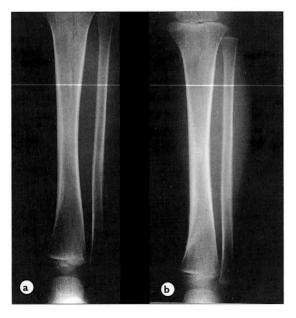

Figure 4.73 a and b
X-ray of the tibia and fibula demonstrating a periosteal reaction on the lateral border of the tibia and a lucent spiral line over the distal end of the tibia. The original X-ray (a) of this child was normal. The second X-ray (b) was taken after 2 weeks in plaster and demonstrates typical appearances of a toddler's fracture.

Talar fractures

Two types of talar fracture occur:
- Minor avulsion fractures.
- Fractures to the body of the talus.

Avulsion fractures occur in plantar flexion injuries of the ankle and also some inversion injuries. They are caused by avulsion of the tendinous or ligamentous attachments to the periosteum. They may be associated with a degree of ankle effusion. Most are treated conservatively with a tubular elastic bandage, crutches and early mobilization. Occasionally, they will require pain relief in the form of plaster cast immobilization for 2–3 days. They should be mobilized as early as possible.

Fractures of the body of the talus can be difficult to diagnose. If diagnosed early they should be treated with bed rest and elevation. The degree of swelling can be considerable. Occasionally, these fractures progress to non-union. These cases should all be referred for an orthopedic opinion.

Fractures of other tarsal bones

Fractures of the other tarsal bones are rare. Treatment will be along the same lines as calcaneal and talar injuries. Considerable swelling is an indication to admit, as is pain. Otherwise children can be mobilized in a tubular elastic bandage on crutches and allowed to weight-bear as soon as the pain eases.

Fractures of the metatarsal

Four types of fracture occur in the metatarsal bones:
1. Avulsion fractures of the base of the fifth metatarsal.
2. Fracture of the shaft of the metatarsal.
3. Fracture of the head of the metatarsal.
4. Liz Franc type injury.

Avulsion fractures of the base of the fifth metatarsal (Figure 4.75)

This injury is caused by sudden inversion of the foot, resulting in avulsion of the insertion of the peroneus brevis tendon. Treatment is symptomatic. Most children can be managed with tubular elastic bandages, crutches and mobilization. A firm shoe probably gives as much support as a cast. Some children, with a lower pain threshold, may actually require some immobilization in a cast.

A variation of this injury is the Jones' fracture which is a fracture of the proximal shaft of the fifth metatarsal. This fracture is prone to non-union and should be referred for early orthopedic opinion.

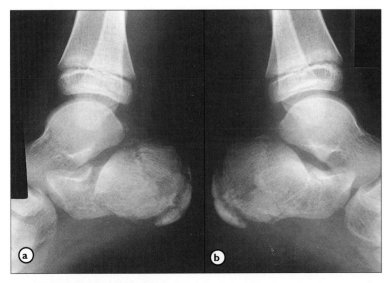

Figure 4.74 a and b
Lateral views of the calcanei of a child who fell on the heels from a height of 15 feet. The X-rays reveal multiple fractures through both calcanei with loss of the normal calcaneal angles.

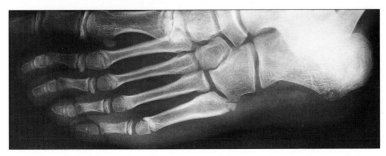

Figure 4.75
Oblique view of the foot in a child sustaining an inversion injury. Note the fracture of the base of the fifth metatarsal with soft tissue swelling along the lateral aspect of the foot.

Fracture of the shaft of the metatarsal

This can either be a fresh injury or a stress injury. Fresh injuries require very little treatment apart from rest. This can be best achieved by keeping the child off the foot for a period of time. Mobilization can be achieved as soon as pain subsides. A firm shoe may give as much support as anything else.

Stress fractures to the metatarsals are rare in childhood (**Figure 4.76**). If suspected clinically, but X-rays are normal, further radiology in 10 days may help. Treatment is by rest initially followed by gradual return to activity as pain allows.

Fractures of the head of the metatarsal

This injury can occur if a child jumps from a height. It can often be missed. Fractures of the metatarsal' heads are often multiple. Admission for elevation is necessary if swelling is marked, otherwise symptomatic treatment is all that is required.

Liz Franc type injury

Liz Franc injuries are mainly soft tissue injuries to the tarso/metatarsal areas of the foot caused by significant hyperflexion around this area. Typically, there will be a history of a fall or jump from a height. There will be marked swelling and tenderness over the forefoot with, often, deceptively normal X-rays. Minor lesions will involve soft tissue injury only. These will need elevation and mobilization if and when, pain permits. Moderate injury will be associated with pain and usually some fractures (often minor) will be present. In these cases, admission for ice treatment and elevation may be required. Major injuries are rare. The main lesions are dislocations at the tarso/metatarsal joints which can easily be missed. Orthopedic opinion is mandatory.

Fracture and dislocation of the toes

Fractures and dislocations of the lateral four toes are rare. Displaced fractures should be reduced as should dislocations of the interphalangeal joints. Buddy strapping is often recommended but is of little benefit—it probably has a placebo effect. The child should be encouraged to mobilize as soon as possible.

Fractures of the great toe are more common. Crush injuries (*see* **Figure 4.49**) are common as are hyperextension injuries. The latter may be caused if the child kicks a hard object 'accidentally'. Unless grossly displaced, no operative treatment is needed. Crutches will help the child to mobilize.

Crush injuries to the foot

The foot is prone to injury from heavy weights being dropped on it. Often no fracture can be seen and the swelling can be considerable (**Figure 4.77**). It is usually prudent to admit these children for at least one night for observation. In this way the foot can be elevated, ice applied and the swelling reduced. The physiotherapist should be consulted at an early stage to supervise treatment and help continue treatment as an outpatient.

SPINAL INJURY

Spinal injury is rare in the pediatric population, particularly in the under-eight age group. This does not mean, however, that it does not occur. The problem of SCIWORA has already been considered earlier in this chapter (*see* **Figure 4.1**).

Spinal fractures in children have the same implications as in adults. The bone lesions will unite well with time but spinal cord lesions will not. The aim of the AED is to identify children at risk of spinal injury either from their history or from any clinical findings made, or both. Once suspected, the child must be offered appropriate protection to prevent further damage or insult to the spinal cord (*see* **Figure 4.3 and 4.12 a and b**).

Both hypoxia and hypovolemia will aggravate spinal cord lesions, so treatment should include full resuscitation along the lines described previously.

Cervical spine lesions are extremely rare in the under-eight age group. Atlanto-axial instability may be a problem for children with Down's syndrome (**Figure 4.78**).

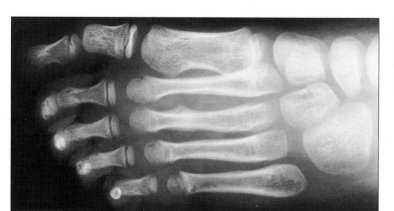

Figure 4.76
Oblique view of the foot showing extensive periosteal reaction and callus formation along the shaft of the third metatarsal. The appearances indicate a healing stress fracture.

Wedge-compression fractures of the dorsal spine are common in falls from a height (**Figure 4.79**). Lumbar spine fractures may be associated with seat belt injuries of the abdomen, particularly when high-speed impacts are involved; lap belts seem to be mostly at fault (**Figures 4.42 and 4.80**).

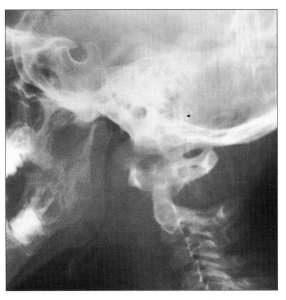

Figure 4.78
Severe cervical spine injury following a road traffic accident. There is dislocation of the C1/C2 vertebrae with widening of the anterior atlanto-axial joint and increased cranio-caudal distance between laminae of C1/C2, with loss of alignment and prevertebral soft tissue swelling.

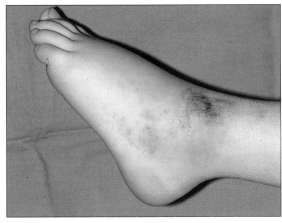

Figure 4.77
Crush injury to the foot. A concrete block has slid down this child's ankle and landed on the foot causing considerable bruising to the dorsum of the foot and an abrasion to the anterior ankle.

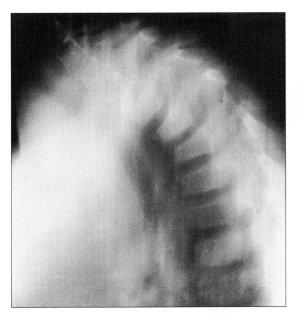

Figure 4.79
X-ray of the lower cervical/ upper thoracic spine showing anterior wedging of the T3/T4 vertebral bodies, following a flexion injury to this area.

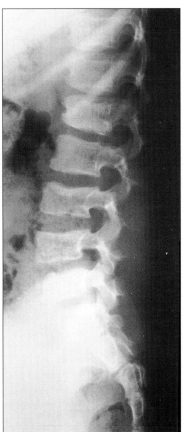

Figure 4.80
Lateral view of the lumbar spine of a 6-year-old child following severe flexion injury to the spine. There is anterior wedging of T12, L1 and loss of height of the L3/L4/L5 vertebral bodies (see also Figure 4.42).

PELVIC FRACTURES

Pelvic fractures are relatively rare in childhood. Several types can occur:

- Fractures of the iliac crest.
- Fractures of the pubic rami.
- Crush fractures.
- Avulsion fractures.

Fractures of the iliac crest

Fractures of the iliac crest usually occur when the child receives a direct blow e.g. from falling onto a hard surface or from a kick. There can be a significant amount of blood lost into the hematoma which is often visible both on the lateral surface (**Figure 4.81**). There is little in the way of treatment that can be offered for these injuries except pain relief and bed rest. If the bleeding is significant, blood transfusion may be indicated.

Fractures of the pubic rami

Again, these usually occur from falls and in childhood are often greenstick in nature. Occasionally, there can be a small degree of separation. If there is any separation at the fracture site one should consider urethral injuries, particularly in males (**Figures 4.40** and **4.82**).

Crush fractures

These are extremely rare but result when a heavy weight rolls over the child, typically in a motor vehicle accident. All pelvic joints are separated and there is often quite severe subluxation or dislocation at the sacroiliac joint. These are serious injuries with severe degrees of hemorrhage and pelvic-structure damage. This will include bladder injuries, urethral injuries or both, with vascular problems giving further complications. These require extensive repair and multidisciplinary treatment (**Figure 4.40**).

Avulsion fractures

Avulsions of muscle origins from the pelvis have been described, particularly of the adductor and quadriceps muscle groups. Most require little more than rest and analgesia but management should be discussed with an orthopedic surgeon.

PATHOLOGICAL FRACTURES

Pathological fractures occur in diseased bone (**Figure 4.83**). Congenital syndromes such as osteogenesis imperfecta and fibrous dysplasia, bone cysts and neoplastic lesions, either primary or secondary, all render bone liable to fracture with minimal trauma. The diagnosis and care of these fractures is beyond the scope of this text. However, the principles of accident and emergency fracture care still hold. The child should be given analgesia, the limb splinted and orthopedic referral made. If neoplasia is suspected then it would be wise to make a referral to a consultant oncologist.

BRUISING AND SOFT TISSUE INJURIES

Most children get bruises every day of their lives. Most are benign but one or two need more extensive treatment and follow-up.

Older boys who receive a kick to the thigh develop what is colloquially known as 'dead leg'. The pain of this is out of all proportion to the apparent nature of the injury. There can be quite considerable swelling of the muscle of the thigh which, if not treated properly, can lead to myositis ossificans (**Figure 4.84**). Early application of ice will reduce the swelling and early active movement of the muscle will reduce the possibility of myositis ossificans. This is best achieved by early referral to a physiotherapist.

Rarely, kicks or blows to the shin, particularly lateral to the medial prominence of the tibia, can result in quite

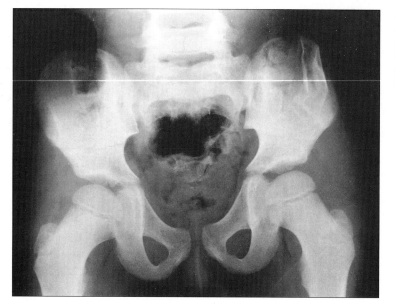

Figure 4.81
Anteroposterior view of the pelvis. This reveals a compression fracture of the left iliac bone. The depressed bone fragments are seen tangentially. There may also be widening of the adjacent sacroiliac joint.

significant hematoma formation. These can be slow to settle and occasionally become infected. If infection supervenes, antibiotics are rarely effective and the child should have the lesion drained surgically. Treated early with physiotherapy the lesion can resolve reasonably quickly (2–3 weeks). This injury can be prevented by advising children participating in contact sports such as hockey, football and rugby to wear shin guards when they are playing.

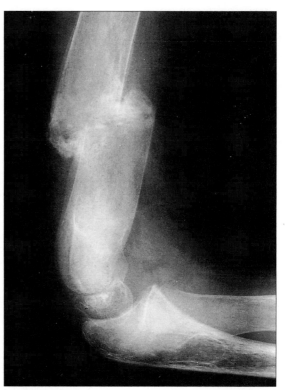

Figure 4.83
An example of pathological fracture of the humerus. The child suffered from fibrous dysplasia. This is manifest by a ground glass appearance of the humerus and proximal radius. The involved bones are expanded with thinning of the cortices. Healing callus is observed at the fracture site.

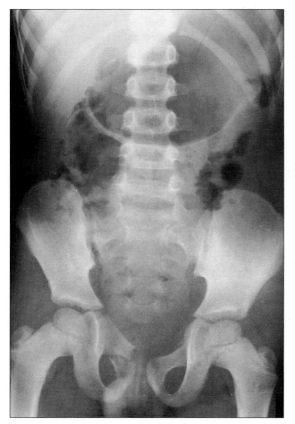

Figure 4.82
Supine view of the abdomen and pelvis in a child suffering abdominal injury following a road traffic accident. The X-ray reveals fractures of both superior pubic rami, widening of the right sacroiliac joint and a fracture of the left iliac bone. Computerized tomography (CT) scanning would show the position and extent of the fractures more accurately. Note also the acute gastric dilation.

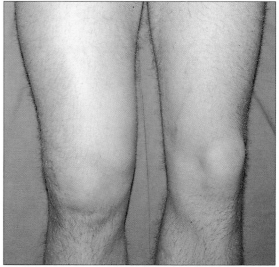

Figure 4.84
This boy received a kick to the right thigh during a game of football. There is considerable increase in size of the thigh due to bleeding in the muscle.

HAND INJURIES

Hand injuries account for approximately 6% of all traumatic injuries in children. As with other aspects of pediatric trauma, blunt injury predominates. The correct management of all hand injuries requires a detailed history, careful examination, judicious investigation and accurate management. Wounds and fractures of the hand heal very quickly making the latter point very important.

FINGERTIP INJURY

Several hundred children each year catch their fingers in a door resulting in damage to the tip of the finger.

Three broad categories of injury occur, any of which can be associated with underlying fracture of the distal phalanx:

1. Avulsion of the nail with laceration to the nail bed.
2. Partial amputation.
3. Subungual hematoma.

When present, the fracture is an open fracture and should be treated as such.

NAIL AVULSION

Nail avulsion can be partial or complete (**Figure 4.85**) with complete avulsion being a rarer entity in our experience. The nail bed should be repaired and tissues approximated. The nail should be repositioned accurately and the wound held firmly with sutures. This will often require a full anesthetic in the younger child in whom cooperation may be lacking.

PARTIAL AMPUTATION

Usually only part of the terminal tuft is amputated together with a varying degree of the pulp. These injuries should

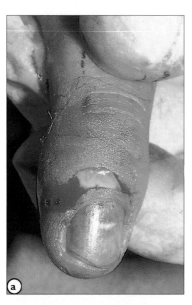
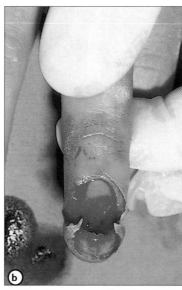

Figure 4.85 a and b
Fingertip injuries with partial (a) and complete (b) nail avulsion. Figure (b) shows the sort of damage that can be done to the nail bed. Similar damage is probably present in (a) but is masked by the nail only being partially avulsed.

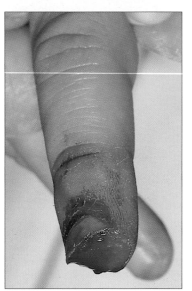

Figure 4.86
Amputation of the finger tip. The tuft of the terminal phalanx is usually exposed.

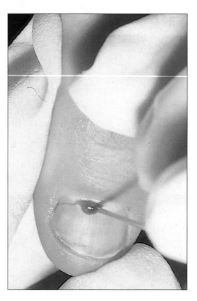

Figure 4.87
Subungual hematoma. This has been drained with a hypodermic needle. A small amount of serosanguineous fluid has been released.

be discussed with a plastic surgeon who can decide further treatment (**Figure 4.86**). Many children with this type of injury will need little more than expectant care.

SUBUNGUAL HEMATOMA

Subungual hematoma is a painful condition related to other types of fingertip injury (**Figure 4.87**). More usually it is caused by a direct blow to either the finger or toe. Bleeding occurs under the nail, building pressure which causes pain.

On presentation, the child should be given analgesia, if required, and sent for an X-ray. The nail should be trephinated to release blood. If the X-ray reveals that a fracture is present the child should be prescribed antibiotics after the hematoma has been trephined. If no fracture is present antibiotics are not indicated.

Almost certainly the nail will be lost and the parents will need to be counseled to this effect. There will often be concern about the regrowth of the nail. While most heal and develop normally, a small number will give problems usually due to damage to the germinal matrix. It is not possible to say at the outset which way any particular nail will develop.

DEGLOVING INJURY

Hands can get trapped in various devices which rotate and traction the skin on the hand or finger (**Figure 4.88**). Occasionally, a ring can get caught dragging the skin with it. The tissue damage is often greater than anticipated and in many cases amputation will be the only option despite the best efforts of the surgical team. Treatment in the AED

will consist of providing analgesia (this is a perfect example of a strong opiate being needed to help allay anxiety as well as providing analgesia), keeping the wound covered and the hand splinted. Radiographs are necessary to help assess the extent of bone trauma. The child should be referred urgently to the Hand Service.

MALLET FINGER

Mallet finger is caused by the sudden flexion of the terminal phalanx while it is being held in extension. Two mechanisms exist for the development of this deformity:
1. Avulsion of the extensor tendon.
2. Fracture through the proximal epiphysis.

In children, this injury is usually the result of a fracture through the proximal epiphysis of the distal phalanx (**Figure 4.89 a**). This injury is not always visible on initial presentation but should be suspected in all injuries to the terminal phalanx.

Treatment is with a mallet extension splint (**Figure 4.89 b**). Many commercial forms exist on the market, only some of which are suitably sized for children. The splint is worn continuously for several weeks, ideally without being changed. This can be difficult to achieve in active children!

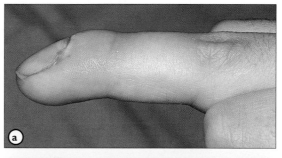

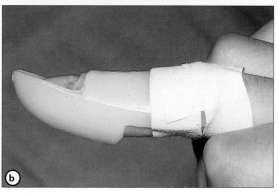

Figure 4.89 a and b
Mallet finger. (a) Typical downward droop of a mallet deformity associated with fracture to the epiphyseal plate of the terminal phalanx. (b) The finger placed in a mallet extension splint. The splint while slightly too big is bringing the distal phalynx into extension and will treat the lesion effectively.

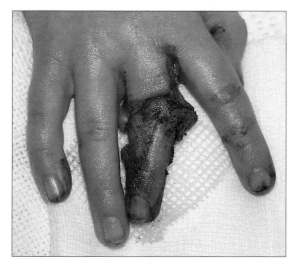

Figure 4.88
Significant degloving injury to the middle finger. This finger was caught in a door when the child was running. There is little hope of salvaging this injury.

VOLAR PLATE INJURY

This is quite a common injury in childhood (**Figure 4.90**). The mechanism is that of forced extension at the proximal interphalangeal joint with the finger held in flexion. This action stresses the insertion of the flexor tendon to the volar aspect of the middle phalanx. Possible injury ranges from a minor avulsion of the tendinous insertion to avulsion of a fragment of cartilage and/or bone. X-rays seldom show any lesion apart from, occasionally, a small avulsed bone fragment. This is best seen on a true lateral view of the joint. Clinically, the joint will be swollen and thickened. Tenderness will be maximal on the volar surface. Movements are painful.

Treatment is by neighbor strapping for 4–5 days and review at this stage (**Figure 4.91**). Movement and function should be assessed. Failure to achieve reasonable function, i.e. almost full flexion and extension, leads to a referral to the physiotherapy department. Virtually all children will have full function restored after several weeks. The finger may remain swollen for a considerable time and the parents should be advised of this at an early stage.

FINGER FRACTURES

Apart from injuries mentioned above, three sites for fracture are common:
1. Fractures to the base of the proximal phalanx.
2. Fractures to the condyle of the middle phalanx.
3. Spiral fracture of the shaft of either the middle or proximal phalanx.

With all of these fracture sites it is important to assess the degree of rotation and deviation (**Figure 4.92**). If the finger is straight and no rotation is present, most injuries of this kind will settle with simple strapping. Any rotational or lateral deformity must be corrected using appropriate analgesia/anesthesia.

THUMB INJURIES

The thumb is prone to the same crush and avulsion injuries as other digits. In addition, the proximal phalanx is susceptible to abduction forces which either stress the ulnar collateral ligaments (gamekeeper's or skier's thumb) in the older child, or the epiphysis in the younger child (**Figure 4.93**). In the case of the latter injury, X-rays are often unhelpful and the injury will be diagnosed on clinical grounds alone. Most of these injuries are quite painful and will benefit from a short period of immobilization in a short plaster cast. Removal at 7–10 days will allow active mobilization to take place.

Children can sustain a fracture at the lower end of the metacarpal which does not affect the joint. This latter injury usually only requires a plaster cast for comfort for 10–14 days.

FRACTURES TO THE METACARPALS

Fractures to the metacarpals are quite common in boys, often as a result of pugilism. Two broad categories of fractures exist:
1. Fractures to the head and neck of the metacarpal (**Figure 4.94**).
2. Undisplaced spiral fractures to the shafts (**Figure 4.96**).

Fractures to the necks of the metacarpals can be quite subtle and are often difficult to spot on X-ray. They are

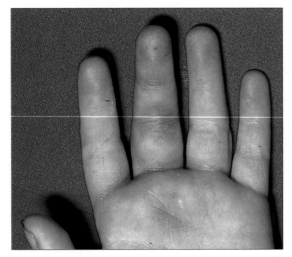

Figure 4.90
Volar plate injury. Marked bruising is present around the proximal interphalangeal joint of the middle finger. While bruising is present from the metacarpal heads to the distal interphalangeal joint, maximum tenderness is elicited over the volar surface of the proximal interphalyngeal joint.

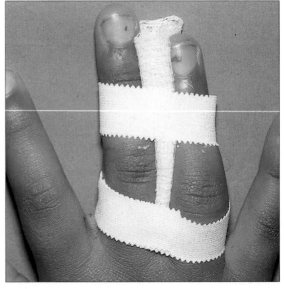

Figure 4.91
Finger strapping. This type of strapping is variably called 'neighbor strapping', 'buddy' strapping or 'garter' strapping.

often Salter–Harris type II fractures into the distal metacarpal epiphysis. Clinically, the knuckle may be slightly depressed in relation to the adjacent knuckles and also when compared to the knuckles on the other hand. The metacarpals most often affected are the fifth (little) finger metacarpal and the second (index) finger metacarpal.

All that is required is symptomatic treatment. The application of a volar splint for 5–7 days gives pain relief and restricts movement allowing healing to take place.

Spiral fractures of the metacarpal shaft are well splinted by the adjacent intra-osseous muscles. Healing usually takes place over a period of 2–3 weeks and again all that is required is splinting in a volar splint.

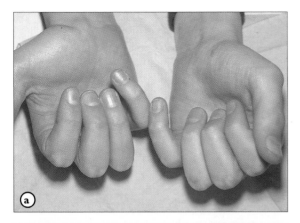

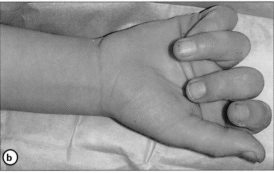

Figure 4.92 a and b
Fracture of the proximal phalanx with rotatory deformity. (a) Fracture to the left little finger with rotation of the little finger away from the other fingers. (b) Fracture of the right little finger with rotation of the finger under the other fingers. Both of these deformities need to be corrected by manipulation.

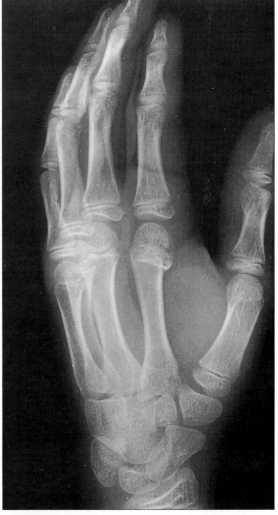

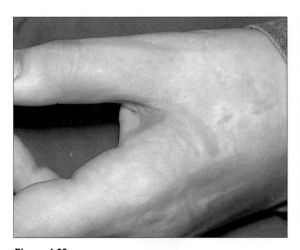

Figure 4.93
Skier's thumb. Bruising and swelling are noted over the base of the thumb on the ulnar border just above the web space. This injury used to be known as gamekeeper's thumb, but in modern society catching rabbits has been superseded by skiing.

Figure 4.94
An oblique X-ray of the hand demonstrating a Salter–Harris type II fracture of the neck of the second metacarpal which shows impaction.

All metacarpal fractures heal with prominent callus formation which is easily palpable on the back of the hand. This gives rise to great concern among parents who should be reassured that this is normal and is part of the healing process (**Figure 4.95**).

Once volar splints are removed the child should be referred to physiotherapy so that active movements can be regained as soon as possible.

CARPAL BONE FRACTURES

Carpal bone fractures are much less common in children than in adults (**Figure 4.96**). Most require simple treatment with immobilization in a volar slab for 5–7 days. Adequate splintage will reduce pain.

SCAPHOID FRACTURES

Injuries to the carpal scaphoid are relatively rare (**Figure 4.97**). Many children will present with pain in the

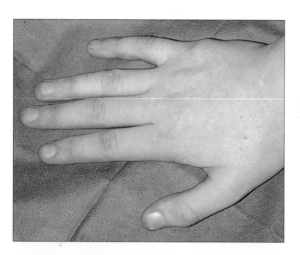

Figure 4.95
Fracture of the fifth metacarpal head. This child is now 3 weeks postinjury. Swelling is noted over the dorsum of the metacarpal head at the fifth finger. Almost full extension is present and he has no functional deficit. This should remodel with time.

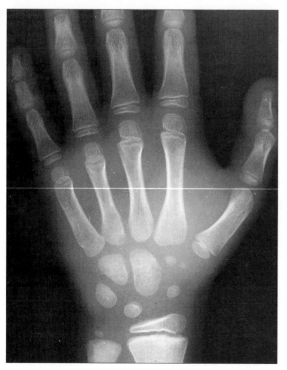

Figure 4.96
Anteroposterior view of the hand. The X-ray reveals transverse fractures through the bodies of the capitate and hamate. There are also fractures of the 2nd and 3rd metacarpals.

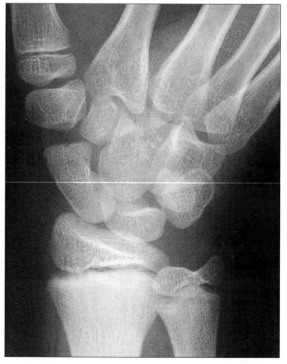

Figure 4.97
X-ray of the wrist demonstrating a fracture of the distal pole of the scaphoid.

anatomical snuff box following a fall on to the hand. Most will have soft tissue injury only. Fractures are more common in the peri-adolescent child although younger children are not immune. As in adults, fractures can occur in the following areas:

- Distal pole.
- Waist.
- Proximal pole.
- Tuberosity.

All fractures should be treated in a plaster and referred for orthopedic follow-up. Suspected fractures (i.e. clinically tender in the anatomic snuff box but no fracture on plain X-rays) should be protected for up to 10 days in a cast for pain relief. At 10 days the cast can be removed and a further X-ray taken. At this stage, if the fracture is confirmed, the child should remain in a cast and be followed-up by the orthopedic service. If no fracture is identified at this stage it is advisable to mobilize the hand as soon as possible at physiotherapy.

Ultrasonic evaluation of the scaphoid area can help identify soft tissue injury from fracture. This technique is not fully proven and more research is needed before it can be recommended fully.

Fractures of the tuberosity of the scaphoid require only short-term splintage for pain relief and then active mobilization. There is no risk of avascular necrosis with this injury.

SCAPHOLUNATE SUBLUXATION

This injury is probably much more common than suspected. A large number of children will present with pain in and around the scaphoid and lunate without evidence of fracture on plain X-rays. These children often have considerable swelling in keeping with soft tissue injury. The ideal treatment for this injury has not yet been elucidated. One approach is to immobilize the child in a wrist splint for several days for pain relief and to actively mobilize the wrist with physiotherapy.

DISLOCATIONS

Dislocation of the fingers is a reasonably common occurrence, either at the metacarpophalangeal joint of the thumb or the interphalangeal joints of the fingers (**Figure 4.98**). Dislocation of the metacarpophalangeal joints is much rarer, and also very difficult to reduce.

The child will present with a deformed finger or thumb following an injury. While it is tempting to reduce the deformity at once it is prudent to wait until X-rays have been obtained. These should be scrutinized for fractures to the epiphyses or interphalangeal fragments. If none are present the dislocation can be reduced using either a ring block, nitrous oxide sedation or both. Occasionally, children will need general anesthesia. After reduction, X-rays should be taken to confirm that the joint has been anatomically aligned and no fractures are present as above. Adequate analgesia should be prescribed and the child referred to the usual follow-up clinics. It is adequate to splint fingers in neighbor strapping, and thumbs in a short scaphoid cast. The latter should be well padded as swelling can be considerable.

SOFT TISSUE INJURIES OF THE HAND
TENDON INJURIES

Tendon injuries of the hand are relatively rare in childhood. Causes include slicing injuries with sharp knives or penetrating injuries sustained in falls on sharp objects, particularly glass. Changes in the composition of glass in buildings in the UK have reduced the incidence of these injuries substantially.

Tendon injuries are difficult to detect in small children. Older children are more cooperative which makes examination easier. Even in these circumstances, movements are restricted by pain, making full assessment difficult.

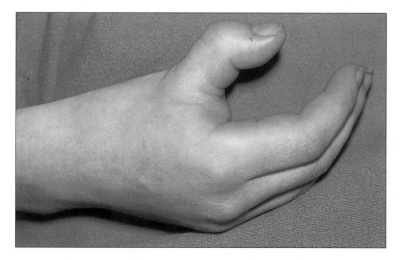

Figure 4.98
Dislocation of the thumb metacarpophalangeal joint.

Approach to tendon injuries in children

The history of the injury is of utmost importance. Once a history of penetrating or wounding with a sharp object is established the possibility of deep-structure damage has to be considered. A full neurovascular assessment of the digits distal to the wound must be made. Radiographs should be taken. If there is either a foreign body visible on the X-rays or tendon injury cannot be confidently excluded, on the basis of clinical examination, the child must be referred to a plastic surgeon/hand surgeon for exploration of the wound (**Figures 4.99 and 4.100**).

There is little place for the enthusiastic amateur in dealing with pediatric tendon injuries.

DIGITAL NERVE INJURIES

The same rules apply to the management of digital nerve injuries as apply to tendon injuries. If there is any doubt about the viability of the nerve distal to a wound, the wound should be explored by those capable of repairing digital nerves under magnification. There is little chance that this can be done effectively in the AED (**Figure 4.101**).

A general approach to the management of wounds can be found later in the chapter.

FACIAL TRAUMA

Facial trauma is common in childhood and is often associated with head injury. Injuries are usually soft tissue in nature with underlying fracture being rare, particularly when compared to the incidence of fracture in the adult population. The incidence of facial skeleton injury increases with age. This may be partly explained by older children, especially boys, engaging in activities which lead to facial injury more frequently!

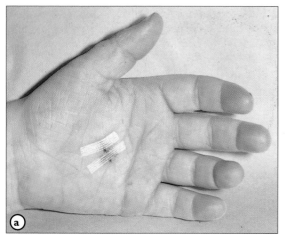
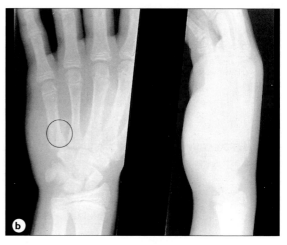

Figure 4.99 a and b
Foreign body deep to the palm. (a) An innocuous wound to the palm following a fall on glass. The wound was not X-rayed initially and the child presented 36 hours after the wound complaining of pain on moving his fingers; (b) X-ray at this stage revealed a deep rooted foreign body.

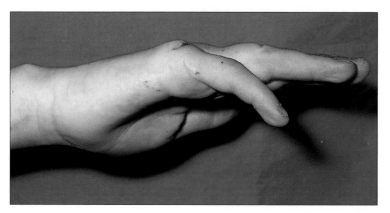

Figure 4.100
Lateral view of the hand. A minor wound is noted over the knuckle of the little finger. The child is unable to fully extend the finger, indicating partial tendon damage. This wound should be explored and the tendon repaired. Almost certainly there will be concomitant injury to the metacarpophalyngeal joint which will need attention.

Common injuries to the face include:
- Mandibular fractures.
- 'Guardsman fractures'.
- Malar injury.
- Ocular trauma.
- Nasal fractures.
- Alveolar-ridge fractures.
- Tooth avulsion.
- Facial lacerations.
- Intra-oral lacerations.

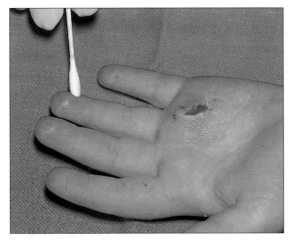

Figure 4.101
Sensation to the digital nerves, distal to the wound, are being tested in the ring finger. As with tendon function, sensory function must be tested distal to all palmar wounds.

MANDIBULAR FRACTURES

Mandibular fractures are sustained when the child receives a direct blow to the bone. Commonly, the bone will fracture in two places. Because the tongue takes origin from the mandible, double fractures can lead to the tongue falling back and subsequent airway obstruction; comatose children laid on their backs are particularly at risk.

Mandibular fractures are often open fractures with communication into the oral cavity leading to infection with oral flora. Prophylactic antibiotics are indicated.

Mandibular fractures should be referred to a maxillofacial surgeon for further management but only after the airway is stabilized (*see* Chapter 1).

GUARDSMAN FRACTURES

This is a variant of the simple mandibular fracture with a characteristic pattern of injury. The child lands heavily on the chin sustaining a wound to the chin. Close examination will lead to the discovery of pain in the temporomandibular joint, particularly on movement. Radiographs often are normal indicating a sprained joint. In some children, fracture of the mandibular condyle or neck may be present. All children with this pattern of injury should be referred to a maxillofacial surgeon for follow-up (**Figure 4.102**).

MALAR INJURY (Figure 4.103)

Direct blows to the orbital region and eye can result in fractures to the underlying facial skeleton. 'Blow-out' fractures of the orbital rim are of particular concern. The extra-ocular muscles in the orbital floor may become trapped in the fracture

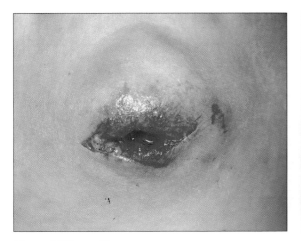

Figure 4.102 a and b
(a) It is common for children to fall on their chin and sustain a laceration. As part of the examination of the wound the child should be asked to open and close the mouth fully. Any pain on full excursion of the mandible at the temporomandibular joint should lead to suspician of a Guardsman's fracture.

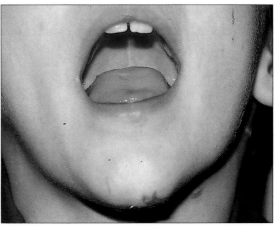

This child has no pain and is able to open his mouth fully, indicating no significant lesion. He did, however, return the next day complaining of pain over the joint which is most likely due to a small hemarthrosis of the joint. Radiographs were normal.

with resultant diplopia on upward gaze. This should be recognized from the outset and the child referred to a facial surgeon. Visual acuity should also be checked and intraocular damage excluded.

OCULAR TRAUMA

One of the more common forms of eye trauma is a scratch to the corneal surface (**Figure 4.104**). Typically, the child is unaware of the cause but presents with severe eye pain and an inability to open the eye. An examination of visual acuity must be made and the eye stained with fluorescein. These injuries usually heal well without any trouble. Ointment containing antibiotic chloramphenicol can help reduce subsequent infection and will lubricate the surface

of the eye. Recent inconclusive reports of aplastic anemia following prolonged use of chloramphenicol have called the use of this antibiotic into question.

Blunt trauma can result in retinal detachment, intraocular hemorrhage and lens subluxation (**Figure 4.105**). All of these will cause some loss of vision but this can be difficult to detect in young children. If in doubt, an ophthalmologist should be consulted. Difficulty may be experienced in examining the eye as local trauma may cause extensive bruising and swelling (**Figure 4.105**). Every effort must be made to examine these traumatized eyes as thoroughly as possible.

Penetrating trauma can be easy to overlook (**Figure 4.106**). Small fragments of metal and stone can easily enter

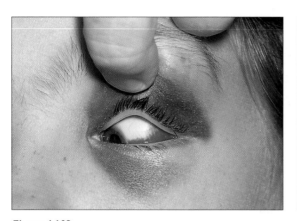

Figure 4.103
This young girl has received a blow to the left side of her face. A subconjunctival hemorrhage is present and she is tender over the orbital margin. Malar fractures are rare in children but should be considered in this pattern of injury.

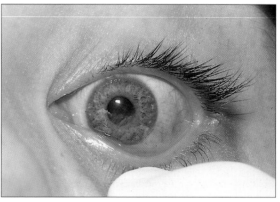

Figure 4.104
Corneal abrasion. This young man has sustained a scratch to his left eye in an accidental collision with another child—he presented with an acutely painful left eye. Fluorescein staining revealed the abrasion in the lower part of the cornea. His visual acuity was normal.

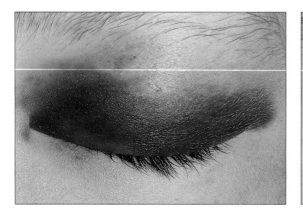

Figure 4.105
Blunt trauma to the left eye. This child received a direct blow to the left eye when he was hit by a stone thrown by another child. On presentation the lid was swollen and tense. In these situations it is important to have a good look at the cornea and intra-ocular structures before the eye becomes too difficult to examine.

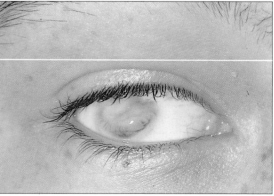

Figure 4.106
Penetrating trauma to the eye is thankfully rare. This child is blind in the right eye following a penetrating injury 2 years previously.

the eye and lodge anywhere within the globe. Larger sharp objects such as darts or knives may leave only the smallest of lesions which are difficult to detect. Clinical acumen and awareness are the keys to diagnosis. Small intra-ocular foreign bodies may show on appropriate X-rays but only if radio-opaque. Ultrasound may help. If penetrating injury is suspected, expert advice must be sought.

NASAL FRACTURES

Nasal fractures occur less frequently in childhood than in adult life. Usually they are the result of a direct blow to the nose. Epistaxis may or may not be present (**Figure 4.107**). Indications to refer for ENT opinion are:

- Deviation visible on inspection.
- Septal hematoma.
- Open fracture.

Difficulty can arise with diagnosis in the presence of soft tissue swelling which can make it difficult to determine whether the nose is deformed or straight. If in doubt, the child should be reviewed after 2 or 3 days when there is still time to organize further management.

ALVEOLAR-RIDGE FRACTURES

Alveolar-ridge fractures are relatively common in the pediatric age group. Children often fall forwards and bang their face on a hard object. Typically, the upper alveolar ridge is damaged but occasionally the lower ridge may be involved (**Figure 4.108**).

The teeth are seen to be pushed back and there will be varying degrees of damage to the gum margins.

Radiographs are seldom helpful though dental films may show some abnormality. This is a clinical diagnosis. If suspected, the child should be referred to a dentist or an oral surgeon for further advice and management.

TOOTH AVULSION

Avulsion of the primary teeth on their own is not really very significant however there can be damage to the alveolar ridge or to the secondary teeth growing below (**Figure 4.109**).

Avulsion of the secondary incisors is a much more serious cosmetic problem. If the tooth can be found it should be brought with the child to hospital in a solution of milk or saliva. Older children may be able to keep the tooth in the buccal sulcus although there is always the possibility of aspiration. It is probably safer to place it in milk. If dental treatment can be obtained readily and easily the child should be immediately referred for further treatment. Otherwise, the tooth should be replaced in the socket and splinted as best one can with whatever is available and dental care obtained as soon as possible.

FACIAL LACERATIONS

Facial lacerations are many and frequent. As with every wound, a history of how the injury was sustained should be obtained. A detailed examination of the wound and underlying structures should be made. The possibility of a foreign body being lodged in the wound should also be borne in mind and X-rays may also be appropriate. The possibility of broken teeth being embedded in the lips must also be considered.

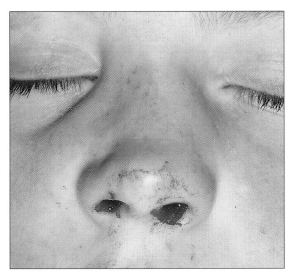

Figure 4.107
Fractured nose with deviation. This young man sustained a blow to the bridge of his nose. The nose is deformed and deviated to the left and will require manipulation.

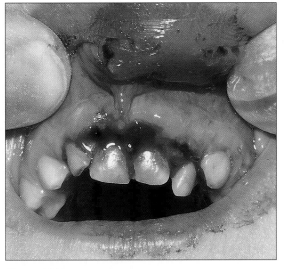

Figure 4.108
This child has fallen forwards injuring his mouth. His primary teeth have been knocked back indicating a fracture of the upper alveolar ridge.

The face is an extremely visible part of the body and consequently all laceration repairs should be done under optimum conditions. Ideally, this means a general anesthetic and the attentions of experienced surgeons.

If it is possible to repair these lacerations in the AED, for instance in older, more cooperative children, then by all means this should be done (**Figure 4.110**). Care should be taken not to use disinfectant solutions round the eyes as these may cause ocular irritation; similarly, if they enter the mouth they can give unpleasant tastes and cause the child to become uncooperative. For this reason all facial lacerations should be washed with normal saline or water.

Deep structures should be repaired with fine catgut and the finest possible sutures applied to the face. Wound opposition should be accurate and all structures should be in their anatomic position, especially eyebrows, nostrils, and lips (**Figure 4.138**).

INTRA-ORAL LACERATIONS

Two broad categories of intra-oral lacerations exist:
1. Penetrating injuries to the palate and soft palate.
2. Biting injuries to the tongue.

PENETRATING INJURIES

Penetrating injuries to the palate and soft palate occur when a child falls with an object already in his or her mouth. There is usually a small amount of bleeding but by the time the child arrives at the AED the foreign body

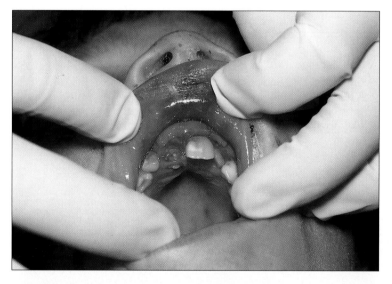

Figure 4.109
This child has fallen forwards avulsing the upper right incisor. Unfortunately, the tooth was lost and so could not be re-implanted.

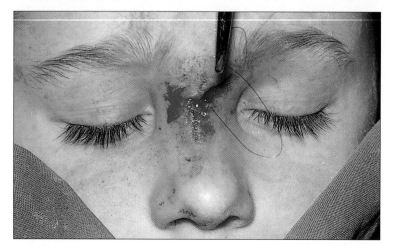

Figure 4.110
This child has sustained a laceration to the bridge of his nose. If this wound is not treated correctly he will be left with a significant cosmetic defect. The wound should be cleansed with saline to avoid clinical irritation to the eyes, which can occur if other disinfectants are used.

has usually been removed (whether rightly or wrongly) and there will be a laceration to the palate (**Figure 4.111 a**).

While the risk of hemorrhage and swelling is slight, it is probably better to admit the child for a period of observation. Surgical edema of the retropharyngeal space can occur. A plastic surgeon should be consulted regarding whether the wound will need further treatment or debridement. This will obviously depend on the nature of the penetrating object and the risk of a retained foreign body (**Figure 4.111 b**).

BITING INJURIES

Children often bite their tongue when they fall and bang their chin, or when they get a blow to their mandible.

Typically, there is a central or lateral flap which usually requires little or no treatment. If there is doubt about the alignment of the tissues, a plastic surgeon should be consulted. Otherwise, these injuries heal spontaneously (**Figure 4.112**).

If no treatment is indicated for intra-oral lacerations, it is important to give the child and parents advice about oral hygiene and the most suitable types of food to eat. It is better to avoid salty and spicy foods which may aggravate intra-oral healing—they may also cause stinging and irritation and cause the child discomfort. In general, sloppy foods, such as scrambled egg, custard and bread, are advisable for the first 24–48 hours following intra-oral laceration. Copious fluids should be given and, if possible, the child's teeth should be cleaned on a regular basis to avoid poor dental hygiene.

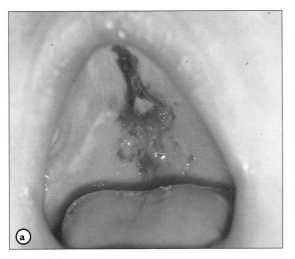

Figure 4.111 a
(a) Laceration to the junction of the hard and soft palate. This child was running with a stick in her mouth. She fell forwards and the stick was jarred backwards causing the laceration.

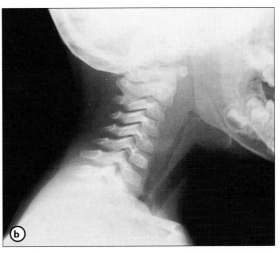

Figure 4.111 b
(b) Lateral view of the neck in a child who had fallen with a pencil in her mouth. There is gas in the retropharyngeal space with a linear lucency following perforation of the pharynx.

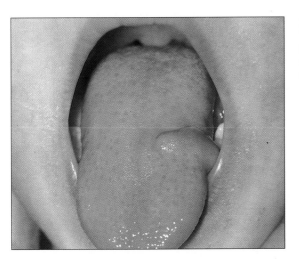

Figure 4.112
This child fell, banging her mandible while her tongue was between her teeth. She sustained a laceration to the left side of her tongue which settled without any treatment. The cosmetic defect at 3 weeks was negligible.

THERMAL INJURY

Thermal injury of all types is a common occurrence in childhood. Despite the ready availability of smoke alarms, education, and prevention initiatives, the mortality and morbidity from fires remains at an unacceptable level. The young child is particularly at risk, with a peak incidence in the under-five age group.

The causes of thermal injury fall into six broad categories:

• Radiation.
• Wet heat.
• Dry heat.
• Electrical burns.
• Chemical burns.
• Smoke inhalation.

RADIATION INJURY (Figure 4.113)

The most common cause of radiation injury is sunburn, with fair-skinned and red-headed children particularly at risk. Mostly this is superficial, with small areas of blistering.

WET HEAT INJURY (Figure 4.114)

Exposure to hot liquids is the most common cause of thermal injury. Hot baths and freshly-made hot drinks, account for most burns in this category.

DRY HEAT INJURY (Figure 4.115)

Burns will occur when children touch hot objects, are exposed to flames or are close to an explosion.

ELECTRICAL BURNS (Figure 4.116)

Electrical burns occur when the child comes into contact with live electricity. The extent of the injury will depend on the voltage applied and the duration of contact.

CHEMICAL BURNS (FIGURE 4.117)

Children will suffer chemical burns if they either touch or ingest acid, alkaline or corrosive substances. Again, the extent of the burn will depend on the concentration of the substance, its corrosive effect and the duration of contact. These burns must be washed in free-flowing water (e.g. a shower) using a detergent if necessary, paying attention to the 'ABC' of resuscitation as indicated.

SMOKE INHALATION (Figure 4.118)

Exposure to smoke or noxious gaseous agents for a prolonged time can result in inflammatory changes in the lungs with or without absorption of poisonous substances. Death often occurs before the child can be extricated from the toxic atmosphere. Some effects, however, can take several hours to manifest themselves, making observation necessary until the danger has passed.

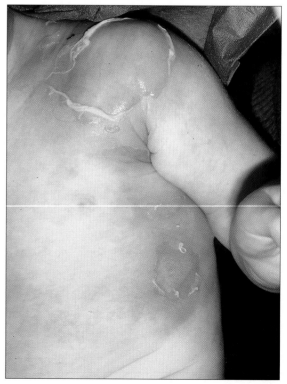

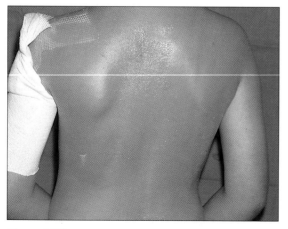

Figure 4.113
Radiation injury. Sunburn is the most common form of radiation injury to children. This child ran around without a shirt for 2 hours on the first sunny day of the summer and sustained quite significant burns to his body.

Figure 4.114
Wet heat injury. This child pulled a freshly made cup of coffee onto her left shoulder and chest.

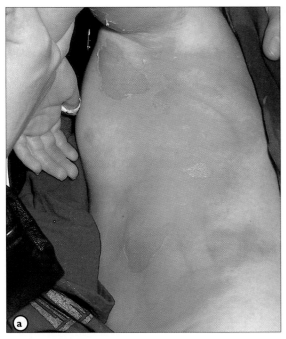
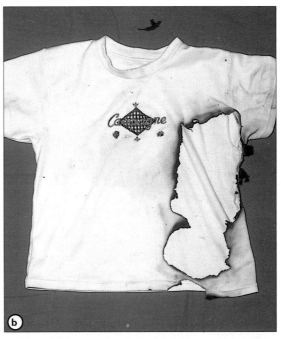

Figure 4.115 a and b
Dry heat injury. (a) shows a child with extensive burns to the left side of her body. She had set fire to her T-shirt (b). The area of the burn is seen to coincide almost exactly with the damage to her T-shirt.

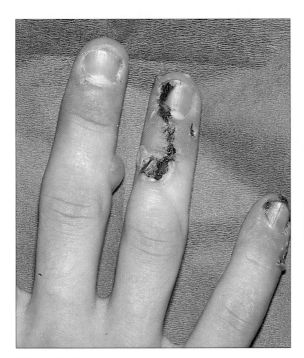

Figure 4.116
Electrical burn to the left ring finger. Note how the burn has affected the adjacent middle and little fingers.

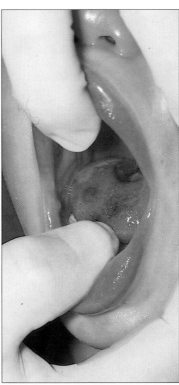

Figure 4.117
Intra-oral chemical burns sustained by a young man who has ingested bleach.

MANAGEMENT OF THERMAL INJURY

When presented with a burned child a doctor should ask the following questions:

- How severe is the burn?
- Does the child need resuscitation?
- Does the child need admission?

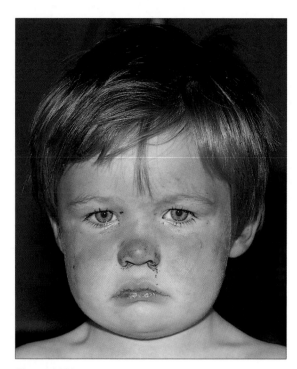

Figure 4.118
Smoke inhalation. The presence of soot on the face around the nose and mouth indicate that this child has been exposed to considerable quantities of smoke. The probability of inhalational injuries and damage to the lung is high.

The answers to these questions provide clues as to how best to manage the burned child successfully.

SEVERITY OF THERMAL INJURY

As a general rule, mortality and morbidity are determined by burn severity. The severity and extent of the burn injury is determined by three factors:

- Depth of the burn.
- Surface area of the burn
- Site of the burn.

BURN DEPTH

Burns can be divided into four categories:

- Superficial.
- Superficial partial thickness.
- Deep partial thickness.
- Full thickness.

Superfical burns (Figure 4.119)

Superficial burns are characterized by the presence of erythema only. They are painful, but heal quickly without residual scarring.

Superfical partial-thickness burns (Figure 4.120)

In this instance there are blisters present, some of which may burst. Where the blisters have burst the underlying tissue will be moist and shiny. Again, these will be painful. Most will heal without any residual scarring unless infection supervenes.

Deep partial-thickness burns (Figure 4.121)

These can be difficult to distinguish from the more superficial type of burn. Again blistering will be present, but the underlying tissue will be less shiny; 'white' areas indicate deep involvement. These will have reduced sensation present. The wounds will be more prone to scarring, a process again aggravated by infection.

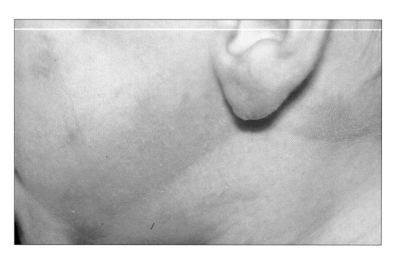

Figure 4.119
Superficial burn to the side of the face in a child who poured a cup of tea onto himself. The skin is red and tender with minimal blistering and the lesion disappeared within 24 hours with no residual scarring.

Full-thickness burns (Figure 4.122)

Here the skin and other tissues will have lost all lividity, have a leathery appearance and be anesthetic. These will usually require surgical treatment, a decision which should be made by a plastic surgeon.

Assessing the depth of a burn is very difficult in the acute stage. It requires experience and practice to gain the necessary expertise. Advice from a senior practitioner should be sought early if there is any doubt.

ASSESSING THE SURFACE AREA OF THE BURN

Several methods exist to assess the surface area of a burn. The palm of the burned child is approximately 1% of the child's surface area. This can then be used to assess the approximate area involved.

More accurate measurements can be made using charts that account for the differing proportions of a child as it grows. The areas can be graphed on to the chart and the areas added up to give a better estimate of the size of the burn (**Figure 4.123**). The burned surface is then expressed as a percentage of total body surface area (TBSA).

Despite these tools, both overestimation and underestimation frequently occur and lead to therapeutic errors, mainly in fluid therapy.

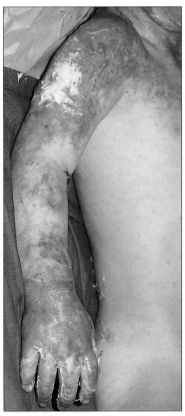

Figure 4.121
Deep partial/almost full-thickness burns to the right arm and hand. Note the lack of vitality in the burnt skin. This child has been transferred from another unit where silver sulphadiazine cream was applied to the upper arm.

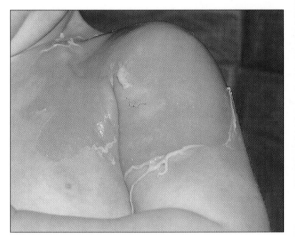

Figure 4.120
Superficial partial-thickness burns. The burned area is moist and shiny where blisters have burst. Whiter (paler) areas represent deeper areas.

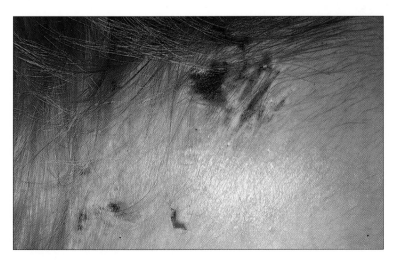

Figure 4.122
Small area of full-thickness burns. Note the leathery appearance and the lack of vitality in the tissue. There was no sensation present.

SITE OF THE BURN

The potential problems caused by burns vary according to the area of the body sustaining the injury. Burns to the perineum and buttocks are more prone to infection (**Figure 4.124**). Burns to the hand and flexor creases of joints may lead to contractures. Circumferential burns to a limb may result is ischemia distal to the burn (**Figure 4.125**). Circumferential burns to the chest can cause respiratory compromise will result. In all these circumstances early discussion with a plastic surgeon is advisable.

Swelling may be a problem following burns to the mouth, face, and neck (**Figure 4.126**). Early protection of the airway is a priority in these circumstances.

OUTPATIENT TREATMENT

Outpatient treatment should only be considered if certain criteria are met. These include:
- The burn is <5% of TBSA.
- The burn is not full thickness.
- The burn does not involve a 'difficult area'.
- No complications exist.
- Home circumstances are good.

Outpatient management will consist of oral analgesia, absorbent dressings, and appropriate outpatient review (**Figure 4.127**).

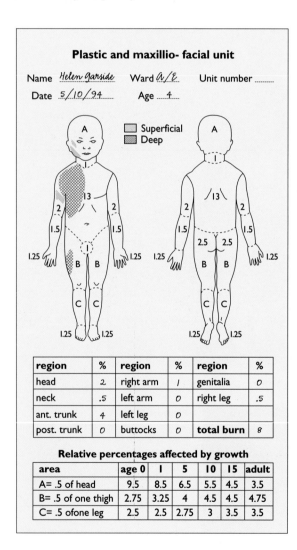

Figure 4.123

Typical burns chart demonstrating graphically the extent of a burn in a small child.

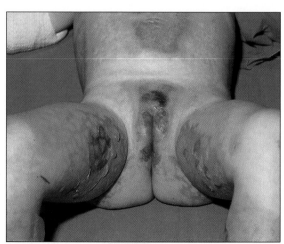

Figure 4.124

This child sustained extensive burns to the perineum, buttocks, inner thighs, and abdomen. She was left in a hot bath with the hot tap running. Injuries around the perineum are very prone to infection. The possibility of non-accidental injury must be considered.

ANALGESIA AND SEDATION

Paracetamol, 15 mg/kg, taken orally together with trimeprazine, 3 mg/kg, is adequate for small burns. Once the burn is dressed the requirement for analgesia is reduced considerably. The dressing is usually tulle gras with a layer of Mupirocin cream as the first layer of the dressing. This is then swathed in absorbent gauze. The entire dressing is secured with tape.

The child is allowed home, with follow-up 7–10 days later. Instructions are given to return if there is seepage through or around the dressing, or if the dressing becomes wet, dirty or smelly. In addition, the child's parents are made aware of the signs of **toxic-shock syndrome**.

Finally, the tetanus status of the child is assessed. Prophylaxis is given according to local guidelines if indicated (*see* **Figure 4.139**).

INPATIENT TREATMENT OF BURNS

A child should be admitted if the criteria detailed previously are not met. Specific criteria for admitting burned children include:
- Burn >5% of TBSA.
- Full-thickness burn.
- Burn affects 'difficult' area.
- Complications present (e.g. smoke inhalation).
- Social circumstances poor.

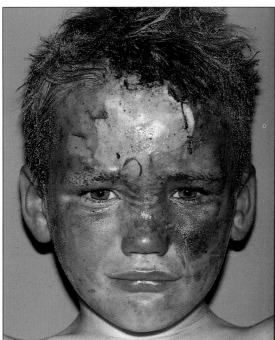

Figure 4.126
This young man has been exposed to a blast injury to his face. His eardrums were normal. He was admitted because of the risk of swelling to his face and airway with potential airway obstruction.

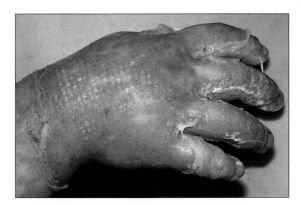

Figure 4.125
This child has extensive burns to the hand. Considerable swelling is already present. These burns need to be managed with great skill and expertise.

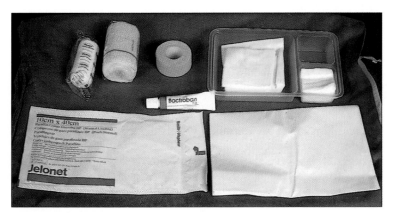

Figure 4.127
Prior to dressing a burn, all equipment should be readily to hand. The burn should be dressed with tulle gras covered with mupirocin cream with layers of absorbent gauze over this. The dressing should be held in place with a clean bandage firmly secured so that it will not fall off.

Once assessed as needing admission for other than social reasons the child should receive parenteral analgesia (morphine 0.1 mg/kg under 1 year of age, 0.2 mg/kg over 1 year of age). The wound should be dressed according to local protocols. Some centers prefer to nurse these wounds open in a warm cubicle.

Again, the tetanus immune status of the child should be assessed and treated appropriately. Fluids may be given orally.

RESUSCITATION IN CHILDREN WITH BURN INJURIES
Resuscitation will be required in a few children who meet the following criteria:
- Burn covers >10% of TBSA.
- Airway at risk.
- Other complications present.

BURN >10% OF TBSA
If the burn is greater than 10% of TBSA, intravenous fluid resuscitation is mandatory. There is debate as to which type of fluid colloid or crystalloid is used. In Britain, the fluid is given as plasma protein according to the Muir and Barclay formula:

$$\text{Volume of plasma in first 4 hours following burn} = \frac{\text{Weight of child (in kgs)} \times \text{Burn surface area (\%)}}{2}$$

This should be calculated from the time of the injury and should be in addition to the maintenance fluids.

The aim is to have a urine output of 1–2 ml/kg/24 hours.

AIRWAY AT RISK
The airway will be at risk if there are burns to the face, neck, mouth or pharynx. Small children who drink hot liquids, especially if heated in a microwave are particularly at risk. Early intubation needs to be considered in all these situations. The airway is also at risk following smoke inhalation (**Figures 4.118 and 4.126**).

SMOKE INHALATION
Smoke inhalation is a complicated entity. Several components contribute to this:
- Irritant action of the smoke particles.
- Toxic effect of hydrocarbons in the smoke.
- Carbon monoxide poisoning.
- Cyanide poisoning.

It is signalled by soot and carbon deposits around the nose and nasopharynx. Other clues include a dry cough, hoarseness or black sputum.

If smoke inhalation is suspected, **humidified** oxygen must be administered to the child urgently. Blood samples should be sent to the laboratory for carbon monoxide

analysis and arterial blood-gas analysis. Blood-gas analysis may show no abnormality early in the process but is a useful baseline.

If significant smoke inhalation has occurred intubation, respiratory support and bronchial lavage may be required. Treatment for carbon monoxide and cyanide poisoning may also be necessary.

Carbon monoxide poisoning
The classic clinical picture of a child with carbon monoxide poisoning having a cherry-red appearance is not always present. Blood carboxyhemoglobin levels are the best way to detect toxic levels of carbon monoxide. Care must be taken to relate the level measured to the time of exposure and the treatment given. Treatment will depend on the levels of carboxyhemoglobin measured and the level of consciousness of the child.

Carboxyhemoglobin levels of less than 10% are probably safe. At levels greater than this symptoms become more likely. Patients with levels greater than 10% should receive oxygen at the highest concentration available by mask. With levels above 30%, significant exposure to smoke is likely to have occurred and 100% oxygen should be administered. This may require intubation. At this level, if confusion or coma are present, treatment with hyperbaric oxygen should be seriously considered.

Cyanide poisoning
Cardiac arrest following smoke inhalation is usually fatal. Normal cardiac arrest procedures should be followed (*see* Chapter 2) but early treatment with **cobalt edetate** should be instigated. This is a specific cyanide antidote with a faster action than sodium nitrite and thiosulphate combination. Cobalt edetate should only be given in cardiac arrest where cyanide poisoning is suspected as it is in itself toxic in the absence of cyanide.

Cyanide poisoning is extremely difficult to diagnose clinically. Cyanide levels are often difficult to obtain from the laboratory service. One method for determining cyanide poisoning is to measure arterial and venous blood gases. If there is a low arterial-venous oxygen difference then cyanide poisoning can be strongly suspected.

OTHER COMPLICATIONS

HYPOTHERMIA
Children exposed to the elements are prone to hypothermia and this tendency is aggravated in burn injury. The skin is an effective thermoregulatory organ, and thermoregulatory loss is proportional to skin damage. In addition, the need to undress the child and the effects of cooling fluids, administered as a first aid measure, combine to make the potential for heat loss considerable. Care should be taken to keep the child dry and warm, ideally in a dedicated environment.

TOXIC SHOCK SYNDROME

Toxic-shock syndrome is a serious condition caused by *Staphylococcus aureus* toxin. While it can follow any break in the epithelial surface, children with burns are particularly prone to this. Any size of burn can be involved and small burns are not immune. A few days after the burn has been sustained the child becomes unwell with systemic illness, pyrexia and rash. There may or may not be associated nausea, vomiting and diarrhea. Mirpirocin dressings and/or flucloxacillin may act as prophylaxis.

The child should be resuscitated as required and admitted for intravenous antibiotic therapy. Blood cultures and wound swabs should be taken if possible before starting antibiotic therapy. Even if treated promptly the condition can prove fatal. A high degree of awareness, therefore, is necessary in all children following a burn injury.

WOUND CARE

Wound management is an important aspect of accident and emergency care. Children pose difficult problems in wound management, particularly in terms of sedation. It should be remembered that wounds presenting to the AED are not the same as surgical wounds created in the operating theatre.

Wounds can be caused by any number of objects all capable of inflicting differing types of injury. Wound management will be best facilitated by adhering to a systematic approach (**Figure 4.128**).

IS THERE ASSOCIATED INJURY?

This question should be approached from two angles:
1. Is there a life- or limb-threatening injury elsewhere which takes priority?
2. Is there an injury associated with the wound that needs treatment, for example, arterial bleeding or underlying fracture?

Only if the answer is 'no' to each of these questions should further treatment of the wound be carried out. Life threatening injuries should be treated as described in Chapter 1. Bleeding should be stopped with pressure and obvious fractures splinted and treated as described previously in this chapter.

HOW HAS IT BEEN CAUSED?

As with all aspects of medicine, a detailed history is essential. Knowledge of the wounding agent and the force applied may influence treatment. This is particularly so with penetrating injury when deeper structures may be involved (**Figure 4.129**). The possibility of a retained foreign body must always be considered. The detection of foreign bodies, that have been retained in the wound, can be very difficult.

Animal and human bites are prone to infection, especially if not recognized early (**Figure 4.130**).

WHAT TYPE OF WOUND IS IT?

When presented with a wound one should determine the type of wound. This will help with general wound management. A typical classification is as follows:
- Abrasion
- Contusion
- Laceration
- Penetrating injury

Questions to ask about any wound

1. Is there any associated injury?
2. How has it been caused?
3. What type of wound is it?
4. Is there a foreign body present?
5. How deep is the wound and what other deep structures may be involved?
6. Is it safe to close the wound immediately?
7. How should the wound best be closed?
8. What dressing should be used?
9. Does the area need immobilisation?
10. Are antibiotics indicated?
11. Is the child tetanus immune?
12. What follow-up is needed?

Figure 4.128
Twelve questions which will faciliate a systematic approach to the care of a wound.

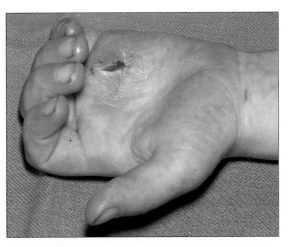

Figure 4.129
Penetrating wound to left palm. Possible structures at risk include the digital nerves, tendons, tendon sheaths and bone. The possiblity of a retained foreign body must be considered.

An abrasion is caused by contact against a rough surface and areas of skin are scraped off. Often particles of grit and dirt are forced into the skin making it difficult to clean fully without general anesthesia. If all particles are not removed, permanent scarring with a tattoo effect will result (**Figure 4.131a**).

A contusion is caused by contact with a blunt object. Not only will the skin be broken but bruised tissue will be present in the vicinity causing additional swelling (**Figure 4.131b**). This will result in swelling proportional to the force applied and the area involved.

Lacerations may be described as **simple** (**Figure 4.131c**) or **complicated** (**Figure 4.131d**).

Simple wounds are caused by sharp instruments such as knives and blades; these cause surgical-type wounds. If caused by falling against objects, such as barbed wire or a tree branch, the wound will be of variable depth and shape leading to dirty, ragged lacerations that can be difficult to treat. Such complicated wounds often require complex plastic surgery to obtain best results.

As the name suggests, penetrating injury is caused by a sharp object penetrating the skin to a variable depth and usually in an unknown direction (**Figure 4.132**). The problem with penetrating injury is that the invisible damage can be out of all proportion to the visible part of the wound and that foreign material can be embedded deeply in the wound (*see* below).

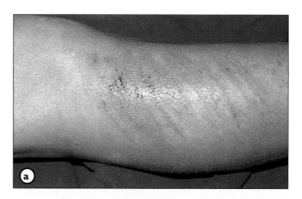

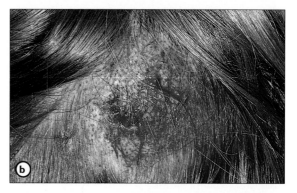

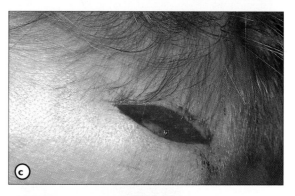

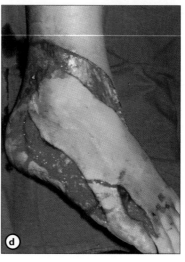

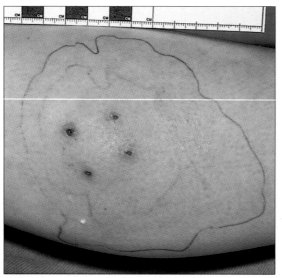

Figure 4.130
Dog bite. Concentric lines demonstrate the original extent of cellulitus and subsequent improvement over time.

Figure 4.131 a–d
a; abrasion
b; contusion
c; simple laceration
d; complicated laceration.

IS THERE A FOREIGN BODY PRESENT?

Some foreign bodies are obvious. The temptation to remove them must be resisted until one is sure that no harm will be done. Foreign bodies are often missed or overlooked. Not all are visible on X-rays, this is particularly the case with wood and plastic. Ultrasound techniques now available make detection easier (**Figure 4.133 a and b**).

Foreign bodies in the foot and hand require full exploration under tourniquet control to be removed. **The temptation to explore these wounds to retrieve foreign bodies under local anesthetic should be resisted.**

HOW DEEP IS THE WOUND?

This can be difficult to assess in children. In particular the presence of deep structure damage can be hard to quantify. Nerve and tendon damage, particularly in the hand, are difficult to detect and full exploration under general anesthetic and tourniquet control is often required. Further problems with assessing the depth of penetrating trauma to the chest and abdomen are often encountered. Again, a full clinical and radiologic assessment will help the diagnostic process.

IS IT SAFE TO CLOSE THE WOUND IMMEDIATELY?

Penetrating wounds and contusions may be better left open unless full cleansing and debridement can be assured.

In the case of penetrating wounds, the possibility of dragging clothing or other particles into the depths of the wound is high (**Figure 4.134**). Infection will supervene if these are not removed. Of more concern is the potential for gas gangrene.

Contusions are associated with extensive tissue bruising which leaves the skin relatively fragile. Associated edema and swelling also reduces the blood flow to the wound which slows healing. The added tension of sutures may aggravate this process.

Exploration, debridement, and treatment of dirty or large wounds takes time and patience to complete (**Figure 4.135**). Few young children will tolerate local anesthetic techniques which makes sedation or general anesthesia necessary. If suitable facilities are available, general anesthesia is best though this will depend on local circumstances.

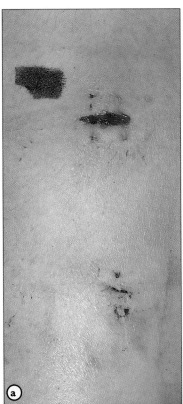

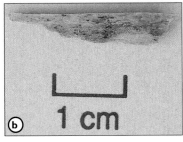

Figure 4.133 a and b
(a) The patient noted a swelling above and medial to the top wound (black mark). (b) The foreign body was subsequently removed. Ultrasound examination revealed this wooden fragment which was not visible on the plain X-ray.

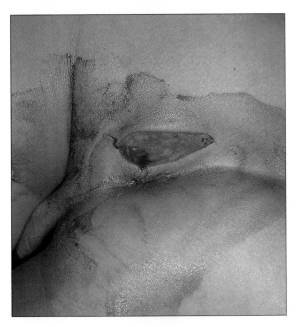

Figure 4.132
This wound was caused when the child sat on broken glass. The possibility of glass remaining in the wound and rectal perforation need to be considered.

HOW SHOULD THE WOUND BE CLOSED?

Several wound closure agents are available: adhesive strips, staples, tissue adhesive (glue) and non-absorbable and absorbable sutures.

Adhesive strips, staples and tissue adhesive are suitable for all simple incised wounds (**Figure 4.136 a and b**). Adhesive strips are not suitable close to joints and other moving areas. They also require a very dry field, as does tissue adhesive. Staples are more robust but require dedicated removal forceps.

If sutures are preferred then non-absorbable sutures are the mainstay in the AED. These can be made from synthetic materials e.g. nylon or natural fibres e.g silk. Nylon sutures will lead to a lower infection rate and better wound appearance (**Figure 4.137**). However, inexperienced operators find these difficult to use, but practice using simulators will make them proficient in handling this type of suture.

Because of the risk of infection, interrupted sutures should be used in preference to subcuticular and continuous sutures. Similarly, closure in layers is not routinely

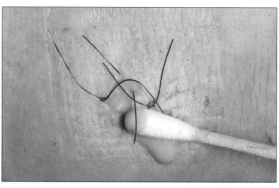

Figure 4.135
A wound which has been sutured without adequate toilet. Frank pus is extruding from the wound and a swab is being taken to aid microbiological diagnosis. After removal of sutures the wound dehisced and organic matter was found in the pre-patellar bursa.

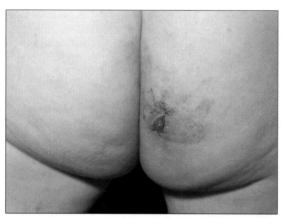

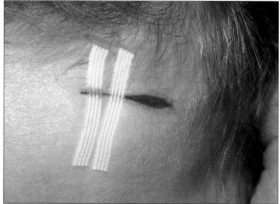

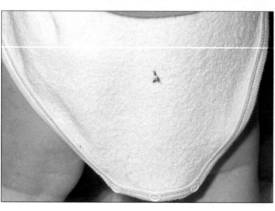

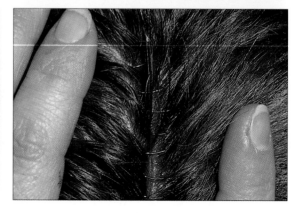

Figure 4.134 a and b
(a) This child fell onto glass sustaining a penetrating injury to the right buttock. (b) Lost threads from the undergarments may well have been dragged into the depths of the wound, making it more prone to infection.

Figure 4.136 a and b
(a) A simple wound being closed with adhesive strips.
(b) A scalp wound closed with metal staples.

recommended for traumatic wounds. These wounds are contaminated for a variable time prior to definitive treatment. Introducing a foreign body in the form of deep sutures adds to the risk of infection which will negate any potential cosmetic benefit derived from suturing in layers (**Figure 4.138**).

It is often difficult to keep children still to enable sutures to be placed with care and precision. As discussed above, sedation or general anesthesia should be used.

WHAT DRESSING SHOULD BE USED?

A decision between using dry dressings or otherwise should be made. Dry dressings are suitable for all simple incised wounds. Abrasions and contusions will need dressings that stick as little as possible; tulle gras is suitable for most wounds of this type. This may be **plain** or impregnated with **antibiotic** or **antiseptic solutions.** Antibiotic or antiseptic creams may also be used.

All other wounds should be dressed with simple dry dressings.

DOES THE AREA NEED IMMOBILIZATION

Wounds over joints may heal more quickly and be less painful if they are splinted **for a few days**. Preventing movement aids the healing process, but may lead to slight muscle loss, especially around the knee.

ARE ANTIBIOTICS INDICATED?

Antibiotics are seldom indicated. They should not be used as a substitute for sloppy surgical technique and incomplete cleaning.

Wounds associated with fractures, deep penetrating wounds and bites may benefit from antibiotic cover. It should be kept in mind that antibiotics in these circumstances are not prophylactic as the potential infecting organisms will already be present.

If antibiotics are thought necessary they should be effective against the organisms most likely to infect the wound. These include *S. aureus* and streptococcal species in most circumstances. Coliforms and anaerobic organisms may predominate in wounds close to the buttocks or perineum. Animal bites, particularly cat bites, may be contaminated with *Pasteurella multocida*.

Another factor in childhood is compliance with medication. Children will usually reject foul-tasting antibiotic mixtures—a factor also important in considering treatment.

IS THE CHILD TETANUS IMMUNE?

Most Western countries have good infant immunization programs, which ensure that children are usually covered against tetanus. However, not all children have been so protected.

TETANUS PROPHYLAXIS

Wounds can be classified into **tetanus prone** (dirty) or otherwise (clean). A tetanus-prone wound is defined as follows:

- >6 hours old before treatment.
- Contaminated with fecal material/foreign bodies.
- Sustained in an area contaminated with manure.
- Significant devitalized tissue present.
- Sustained by a child not immunized.
- Puncture-type wounds.

All wounds should be assessed and classified appropriately. Each wound should receive appropriate cleaning and debridement under suitable anesthesia. Tetanus prophylaxis should be given as determined by the tetanus status of the child and the nature of the wound (**Figure 4.139**).

Children in the UK get a combined tetanus and diphtheria toxoid booster at junior school entry (age 4–6 years). If a child of this age sustains a wound that is considered to need tetanus prophylaxis it is prudent to administer a combined injection of tetanus and diphtheria toxoid in the AED; a second injection against diphtheria will not then be required at a later stage.

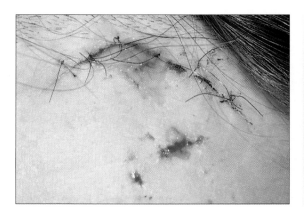

Figure 4.137
A wound closed with fine nylon filament. This will result in a good cosmetic appearance. The smaller wound is awaiting repair.

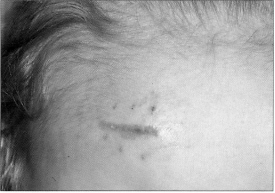

Figure 4.138
A wound poorly closed with thick braided silk suture; the sutures were left too long prior to removal. Almost certainly infection has supervened and this will result in permanent scarring.

WHAT FOLLOW-UP IS NEEDED?

Factors to be considered include dressing changes, wound review and suture removal. These will depend on local policies and practices. As a rule most wounds do not need daily dressings. Parents should leave the AED with a clear idea of what to do to keep the wound clean and dry. They should also be aware of what to do if problems occur.

SPECIAL SITUATIONS

Wounds that require special attention or particular treatment include:

- Wounds in diabetic patients.
- Wounds in children on steroids.
- Needle-stick injuries.

DIABETIC PATIENTS

Diabetic patients are more prone to wound infection than the population at large, especially if control is poor. This in itself does not lead to different treatment methods and the principles of treatment detailed above should be sufficient. Of more concern is the need to check the blood sugar (stick testing is sufficient) and to monitor this more closely than normal. There may be an increased need for insulin which should be discussed with the diabetic team.

PATIENTS ON STEROIDS

Prolonged steroid therapy causes delay in healing and by altering the skin texture can make tissue handling difficult. Sutures may pull out in areas where the steroids have thinned the skin. If in doubt about skin closure in difficult areas, plastic surgeons should be consulted.

NEEDLE-STICK INJURIES

Children often come into contact with discarded needles in the community, the origin of which is unclear. The worry is that the needles will have been used for illegal drug injection and so possibly be contaminated with blood from people infected with human immunodeficiency virus (HIV), hepatitis B, other hepatitis strains or any combination of these. Infection from these sources is an extremely remote possibility, particularly in view of the fact that viruses do not live for any length of time outside the body. However, the theoretical risk, and the worry and concern engendered in parents, requires the situation to be handled with consideration.

The wound should be cleaned and dressed as appropriate. Blood should be taken from the child who has sustained the needle-stick injury—this should be sent for assessment of hepatitis B status. Part of this sample will also be stored for possible further analysis. In the meantime, the child is offered immediate passive (gamma globulin) and active (hepatitis B) vaccine immunization (**Figure 4.140**). Arrangements should be made for the child and family to have counselling at the outpatient HIV clinic where the risks of HIV, hepatitis B and other forms of hepatitis infection will be discussed. HIV testing will not be carried out on the first sample unless counselling has been provided and parents have given fully-informed consent. Further treatment and blood tests will be offered after this. It is usual for an accelerated course of hepatitis B immunization to be offered (after 1 and 2 months following the incident) and accepted. Blood will be drawn after a sufficient time

Figure 4.139

Regimen for tetanus prophylaxis		
Tetanus status	**Clean wound**	**Tetanus prone wound**
Fully immunized or booster <10 years ago	No treatment	No treatment*
Full immunization or booster >10 years	Tetanus toxoid booster**	Tetanus toxoid booster** plus HTIG
Not immunized or doubt about status	Full immunization course	Full immunization course plus HTIG

* If the wound is heavily contaminated or it is nearly 10 years since immunization, a dose of tetanus toxoid should be administered. This also supposes full surgical toilet is performed.

** Adsorbed tetanus vaccine. In children it is desirable to give combined tetanus toxoid and diptheria toxoid to prevent additional single diptheria vaccination subsequently HTIG, Human Tetanus Immunoglobin. This should be administered in a different site to the toxoid.

has elapsed for an antibody response to be raised. The sample can also be sent for further HIV or hepatitis testing if required. There is no evidence to support the use of AZT (zidovudine) in childhood needle-stick injuries.

NON-ACCIDENTAL INJURY

CHILD ABUSE

The total extent of child abuse in the community is unknown. Consequently, the numbers presenting to AEDs are similarly unknown. Child abuse takes many forms which can and do coexist (**Figure 4.141**).

The role of the AED in the management of child abuse is variable. It will depend primarily on the experience and skill of the staff working in the department itself and the roles adopted by senior staff in the department.

Some departments will be the local focus for child abuse investigation. Senior staff within such departments will have expertise and training in the examination of these children and a system of referral will be in place. There are merits to this practice in that the department is open all the time with facilities and staff available.

A child may be referred to these departments by an outside agency (e.g. social services, teacher, police) that has reason to suspect that the child has been abused. They will require a physical examination of the child either to confirm or refute the suspicion. It is desirable that a room, which is comfortable and as non-clinical as possible, be made available. It should be bright and cheery yet have storage space for all the equipment needed for a full forensic examination.

Only a few departments function in this fashion and most of these will be ones which only treat children. Many more departments will refer children suspected of being abused to another team, usually the on-duty pediatricians or the community pediatric team. This team will have the same function as that detailed above.

Alternatively, a child may present to the department with a pattern of injury, radiographic abnormalities or other suspicions which suggest that all is not well.

In this situation, it is vital that the AED staff are all familiar with the patterns of child abuse, the injuries that make one suspicious and other features that may indicate that a child is at risk. Once suspected, there should be a mechanism for referral for further investigation.

PHYSICAL ABUSE

Physical abuse is the most common form of abuse to present to the AED. It is prevalent in the under-five age group, but should be considered at any age.

Diagnosis of physical abuse
Pointers to a diagnosis of physical abuse include:
- Changing history.
- History inconsistent with injury.
- Delay in seeking medical advice.
- Past history of abuse.
- Sibling abused.

Phrases like 'he must have fallen' or 'his older brother hit him' are often clues to the diagnosis. Delay in seeking help should be taken with care as parents will often seek help from pharmacists, neighbors with experience of first aid or other persons. That they did not visit a physician should not necessarily be held against them.

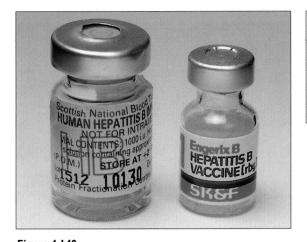

Figure 4.140
Active and passive immunisation are required following needle stick injuries where the origin of the needle is unclear and in human bites where the hepatitis B status of the assilant is either unknown or unclear.

Forms of child abuse
Physical abuse
Sexual abuse
Emotional abuse and neglect
Munchausen-by-proxy

Figure 4.141

Families where abuse has occurred previously are at risk of experiencing abuse again. Siblings of abused children are therefore at risk. Previous knowledge of the family is important, making the role of the social services, general practitioners, and health visitors vital.

Examination of the child who is suspected of being abused is vitally important. The child should be examined from top to toe looking for evidence of injury. Often typical patterns of belt marks (**Figure 4.142**), hand prints (**Figure 4.143**) or cane strokes (**Figure 4.144**) will be visible. Bruises to the ulnar border may indicate defensive activity (**Figure 4.145**). Bruises of different ages can be helpful in diagnosis. However, it can be difficult to age bruising accurately. Injuries visible on plain X-rays are often very good pointers to the presence of non-accidental or repeated injury.

Of particular concern are fractures in the under-one age group. It is rare for these to occur. Any fracture in this age group should be taken seriously. An exception to this is birth trauma which can result in fractures to the femur, chest, arm or clavicle (**Figure 4.146**). **Figures 4.147–4.149** demonstrate typical X-ray findings in non-accidental injury.

Specificity of radiological findings

Lesions can be divided into high-, moderate- or low-specificity as follows:

High specificity:
- Metaphyseal lesions.
- Posterior rib fractures.
- Scapular fractures.
- Spinous process fractures.
- Sternal fractures.

Moderate specificity:
- Multiple fractures, especially bilateral.
- Fractures of different ages.
- Epiphyseal separation.
- Vertebral body fractures and subluxations.
- Digital fractures.

Common, but low-specificity:
- Clavicular fractures.
- Long-bone shaft fractures.
- Linear skull fractures.

Moderate- and low-specificity lesions become high when history of trauma is absent or inconsistent with injuries.

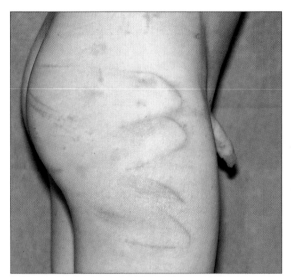

Figure 4.142
This child has been hit at least four times with the end of a belt. The marks are on his right buttock and have been inflicted by a right-handed person.

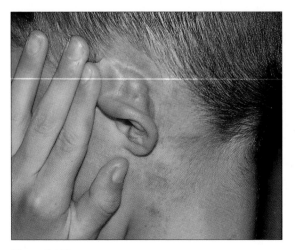

Figure 4.143
This child has been hit on the side of his face by an adult's hand. Imprints of the adult's hand are seen behind the ear over the mastoid region.

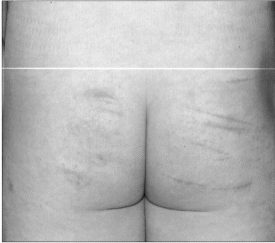

Figure 4.144
This child has been hit with a bamboo cane. The narrow wheals are typical of this type of assault weapon.

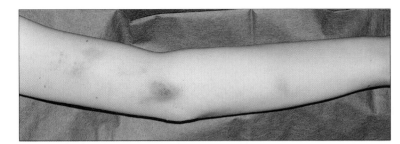

Figure 4.145
Defensive blows over the ulnar border of the right arm. The arm has been placed over the face in an effort to protect the face from blows raining down on it with a broom handle.

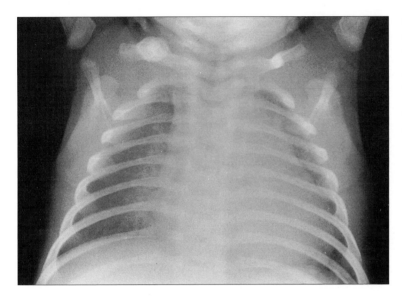

Figure 4.146
Anteroposterior view of the chest of a neonate. There is a healing fracture of the right clavicle. The X-ray reveals the calcifying callus over the middle third. The fracture is at least 3 weeks old and is the result of birth trauma. The child also has a ventricular septal defect manifest by the enlarged heart and increased pulmonary vascularity on the chest X-ray.

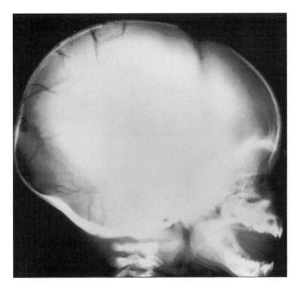

Figure 4.147
Lateral skull X-ray. The X-ray shows multiple fractures in the parietal and occipital bones. This is a case of non-accidental injury.

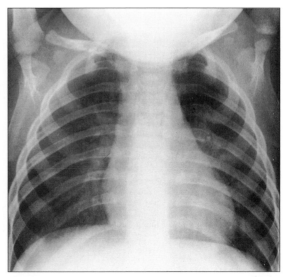

Figure 4.148
Chest X-ray on the same infant as in **Figure 4.147** demonstrating healing fractures of the posterior ends of the left fifth and sixth ribs.

Babies and small children are often shaken violently. This can result in diffuse brain injury with little evidence of external injury to the head. Retinal hemorrhages may be visible on ophthalmoscopy (**Figure 4.150**). If suspected, the child should be examined carefully for signs of finger prints to the trunk and limbs.

Burns are also a feature of child abuse. An accidental burn typically affects the head, face or trunk. Burns which affect the feet (**Figure 4.151**), buttocks (**Figure 4.152**) and dorsum of the hand (**Figure 4.153**) are more likely to be deliberate.

If child abuse is suspected, the child should be examined as detailed above. A clotting screen should be conducted to exclude an underlying bleeding diathesis and radiologic investigation should be carried out to look for other injuries.

At this stage there will be a body of evidence which should be taken as a whole. It should be considered along with a knowledge of the family obtained from the social

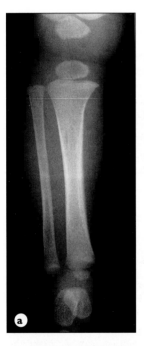
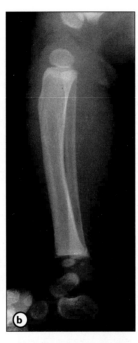
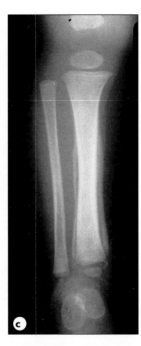

Figure 4.149a–c
(a) Anteroposterior and (b) lateral views of the tibia and fibula in a child having suffered a flail-like injury of the lower leg, following shaking. There are corner fractures involving the distal tibia, best seen on the lateral film. (c) Anteroposterior view of the same leg. This shows extensive healing and periosteal reaction along the tibial shaft 11 days after the initial injury.

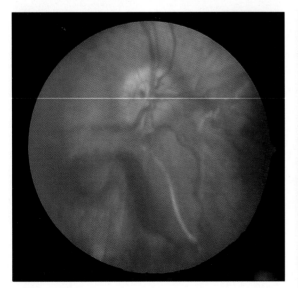

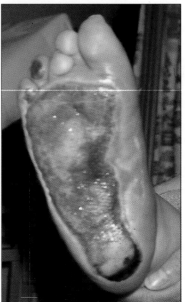

Figure 4.151
Deep burns to the sole of the foot of a child who was deliberately immersed in hot water as a punishment.

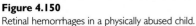

Figure 4.150
Retinal hemorrhages in a physically abused child.

services, health visitors and general practitioners. Three scenarios are then possible (**Figure 4.154**), each with a defined plan of action.

Management of physical abuse

In the case of definite child abuse the situation should be carefully explained to the guardians of the child. Arrangements for the safety of the child are paramount. The child may be admitted to hospital or discharged to foster care. In exceptional cases the child may be allowed home. The latter should only be considered if there is absolute certainty that the child will be safe. Police and social service enquiries will follow as rapidly as possible.

In the event of the evidence from the medical consultation being inconclusive the child should be allowed home with further social work investigation and follow-up. A police investigation will also be necessary. In both proven and inconclusive situations there is a need for a case conference to be called.

Where child abuse is confidently excluded on the basis of medical examination, the guardians should be informed and the situation discussed with them. A normal outcome on this occasion should not lead to any prejudice in the future.

SEXUAL ABUSE

Very occasionally children will make a disclosure to someone in the AED when they have presented for treatment of another problem. Alternatively, a combination of history and physical signs and investigations will lead one to place sexual abuse high on the differential diagnosis. These include:

- Vulval damage/vaginal tears.
- Anal damage either acute or chronic.
- Proven sexually transmitted disease, e.g., gonococcal infection.
- Teenage pregnancy.

Conditions such as anorexia nervosa, bulimia, parasuicide

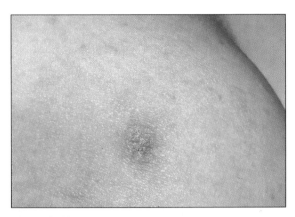

Figure 4.152
Cigarette burn to the buttock of a physically abused child.

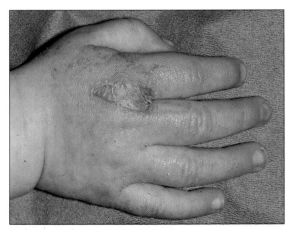

Figure 4.153
Burn to the back of a hand. This child presented with a burn several days after it had been inflicted. When confronted, the child's mother admitted to putting the tip of a hot iron on the back of the child's hand to 'teach her a lesson'. A combination in delay of presentation and the atypical site of the burn aroused suspicions before the mother had admitted causing the burn.

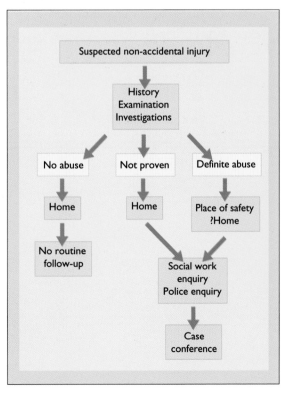

Figure 4.154
Management of non-accidental injury.

and attempted suicide, truanting and antisocial behavior may all follow sexual abuse. Other causes, however, should be excluded first before making a diagnosis in the AED.

There should be well publicised mechanisms within each department, based on local policies and guidelines, to enable these children to obtain appropriate treatment and follow-up.

Very occasionally a child will present having been raped or severely assaulted. In this situation there are three important stages in management.

These are:

1. Resuscitation following the principles described previously.
2. Preservation of evidence wherever possible.
3. Helping the child/family to come to grips with the problem in whatever way possible.

MUNCHAUSEN-BY-PROXY

Again, the incidence of this condition is unknown. Typically, the mother is involved. In this condition the parent deliberately harms the child but seeks medical advice very soon after the insult. Suffocation, factitious hematuria and deliberate poisoning are three of the types of insult that can be administered.

This is a difficult condition to pick up in the AED. First of all a high index of suspicion is needed, but even then it is difficult to believe that a child with apnea attacks is actually being suffocated! Secondly, systems should be developed which will identify not only this type of abuse but also other types of abuse (this is discussed below).

EMOTIONAL ABUSE/NEGLECT

Again, this can be difficult to detect in the AED. Evidence that the child is being abused or neglected, either emotionally or otherwise, may be detected by failure to achieve milestones or neurological regression. Speech delay is common in abused children; it is important to rule out organic causes first. A child may also show a lack of bonding with the parents.

One should be wary of labeling dirty, unkempt children as being neglected. In these children it is more important that one looks at both the relationship between the child and his or her parents.

ACCIDENT AND EMERGENCY SYSTEMS TO DETECT CHILD ABUSE

Within the AED, systems should be established to help detect children who are at risk of abuse. The aim would be to detect frequent attenders or different patterns of attendance.

These systems will include the following:

Computerized records that identify frequent attenders in all children

Once identified these should be audited and discussed with the general practitioner or health visitor who may also have concerns. If further cause for concern is identified then referral to social services should be made.

Computer systems that are able to identify aliases, common addresses or common parents

These may also help in the detection of abuse. It is not unknown for parents to bring children to the AED and use a different surname in an effort to avoid detection. Record linkage and searches using first names, address and post code can help to identify the parents of these children.

All previous clinical notes relating to the child's attendance should be stored in the one place

Ideally, this should include inpatient and outpatient notes. Previous attendances can then be scrutinized and patterns analyzed. Munchausen-by-proxy may be detected in this way. In addition social work presence and good 2-way communication will facilitate good management of abused children.

Chapter FIVE

Surgical and Related Problems of the Child in the Accident and Emergency Department

PEDIATRIC ORTHOPEDICS

Many children present to the AED with acute and sub-acute conditions related to the musculoskeletal system. Many of these will have pathology peculiar to childhood. The purpose of this chapter is to introduce the topic and to provide an approach to the management of these children.

ACUTE HEMATOGENOUS OSTEOMYELITIS

As the name suggests, this condition is different to osteomyelitis associated with open fractures or fixation of closed fractures. While a primary focus of infection may be implicated (for example, a carbuncle) it is not usually possible to identify such a site. While any organism may be the infectious agent the most common is *Staphylococcus aureus*, closely followed by *Streptococcus pyogenes*. Coliforms are common in the neonatal period.

While any bone can be affected, lower limbs are most frequently involved. Osteomyelitis is usually a virulent infection and the child is usually toxic. Typically, the child will present reluctant to use a limb or part of a limb. Pyrexia is usually evident (pyrexia of unknown origin may be due to osteomyelitis, especially in the neonatal period).

Focal signs may be absent in the very early stages but careful palpation of the limb will usually elicit an area of tenderness. Typically, the tender area will be adjacent to an epiphysis. As the disease progresses increased skin temperature, redness and swelling may also be found in this area. Occasionally, a joint effusion may also be present.

Radiographs taken at this stage may show soft tissue swelling and displacement of fat pads. Periosteal and bone changes take up to 10 days to appear in the bone (**Figure 5.1**). Of more use, however, is a full blood count, erythrocyte sedimentation rate (ESR) and C-reactive protein. Typically, the white cell count is raised with neutrophil predominance. The ESR and C-reactive protein are early markers of acute inflammation and will invariably be raised. Ultrasound may reveal periosteal elevation and sub-periosteal abscess at 2–3 days. A positive radioisotope scan may be seen after 12 hours.

The main differential diagnoses will be between cellulitis and septic arthritis.

Management will include siting an intravenous line, taking blood for a full blood count, ESR, blood cultures, and initiating iv antibiotics, for example, flucloxacillin and/or sodium fusidate. Fluid resuscitation may also be

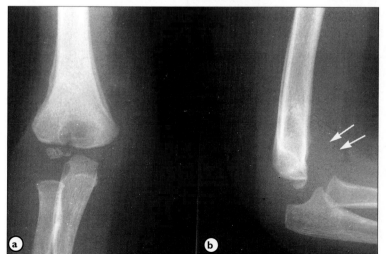

Figure 5.1
(a) Anteroposterior and (b) lateral views of the elbow. There is an ill-defined lytic area involving the distal humerus metaphysis. A destructive area is also seen in the capitellum and there is a healing periosteal reaction along the shaft of the distal humerus. An elbow joint effusion is also present (note the elevated anterior fat pad arrows). The images are of an osteomyelitis of the distal humerus.

required. The limb should be splinted if possible and the child given antipyretics and analgesia as appropriate.

The child should be admitted under the care of an orthopedic surgeon who may consider the therapeutic options of operative versus conservative treatment.

SEPTIC ARTHRITIS

In the case of septic arthritis, the clinical picture is often similar to osteomyelitis and it can be difficult to distinguish between the two clinically; similar organisms are involved. However, *Haemophilus influenzae* will affect about 15% of cases. Hopefully, vaccination will reduce this cause significantly.

The clinical picture and management of this condition are similar to that in osteomyelitis. Children with septic arthritis will have exceptionally painful joint motion. Ultrasound will show joint effusion (**Figure 5.2**). Aspiration of the joint, under aseptic conditions and under general anesthesia, will provide samples for bacteriology, and aid appropriate antibiotic selection. If *H. influenzae* is present on the initial Gram stains, specific therapy can be instituted according to local sensitivities (a varying resistance to ampicillin exists in the community, so treatment should follow local guidelines).

Until direct evidence of the organism is available, either from aspirate or blood culture, the treatment used should be effective against staphylococci, streptococci, and Haemophilus.

Again, the limb should be splinted and the child given analgesia and antipyretics as indicated.

IRRITABLE HIP

This is a generic term which covers a multitude of diagnoses. No child should ever have this as a final diagnosis until many other conditions have been ruled out.

TRANSIENT SYNOVITIS

This is a self-limiting disorder of unknown etiology, more common in males than females. The hip is the most affected joint but the condition can occur in any joint. Typically, the child is aged between 2 and 7 years and presents with a limp of relatively short duration. Pain is not a universal feature. A history of pre-existing viral illness should be sought. A recent upper respiratory tract infection, cold, or mild gastroenteritis is often obtained in the history. The exact relationship between these events is unclear.

Examination will reveal a well child, non-toxic in appearance, and apyrexial. The presence of toxicity or pyrexia should lead one to seek another diagnosis such as osteomyelitis or septic arthritis. Examination of the joint will reveal limitation of movement—the degree of limitation varies from child to child. Movement is often painless, but if painful movement is present it should lead one to exclude sepsis.

It is prudent to examine the rest of the child looking for signs of other pathology. One should palpate the abdomen looking for hepatosplenomegaly, examine the axillae and neck for lymph nodes, and ensure no gross spinal pathology is present. The rest of the limb is also examined to exclude another cause (*see* The Limping Child, page *142*). The child should also be observed walking.

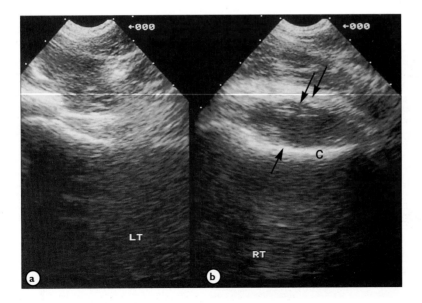

Figure 5.2
Longitudinal ultrasound scan of the hip joints of a child with septic arthritis. The left hip (a) is normal. The right hip (b) shows fluid collection within the joint (short arrows). Note the thickened hip capsule (long arrow). C= cortex of femur.

Appropriate investigation will include a full blood count and ESR or C-reactive protein. Viral titres may be helpful but are not mandatory. Blood cultures should be taken in pyrexial children. Radiographs of the hip are often difficult to interpret for inexperienced doctors. If transient synovitis is present an effusion may be visible. An ultrasound scan of the hip joint will confirm the presence of fluid more effectively.

Management will depend on the history, physical findings and the results of investigations. Children should be admitted for bed rest if:

- There is marked limitation of movement in the joint.
- There is painful joint movement.
- The full blood count or other tests indicate bacterial infection.

If there is concern about parental ability to effect adequate bed rest for the child, admission may also be considered.

Children should be allowed home for bed rest if the joint is painless, the range of movement is good, the child is apyrexial and non-toxic and the blood parameters are normal or compatible with viral infection. The parents are advised that the child should rest as much as possible and stay away from school. Review is organized after 5–7 days but parents are advised to bring the child back if there is any worsening of the condition, particularly if signs of infection occur.

It should also be borne in mind that 5–7% of children with transient synovitis will develop Perthes' disease. The unlucky ones are not easily identified on initial presentation.

MISSED CONGENITAL DISLOCATION OF THE HIP

Limp, or more precisely a peculiar gait, can often be the first indication that a missed congenital dislocated hip is present. The child is usually under 2 years of age. Examination can be very difficult. Examination of the child walking may show a typical Trendelenberg gait. A X-ray is necessary to confirm the diagnosis. If dislocation is present, the child should be referred to an orthopedic surgeon.

PERTHES' DISEASE (Figure 5.3)

Perthes' disease is a condition of unknown etiology affecting children in the 2–8-year age group. Often the child has an intermittent limp and may have a history of transient synovitis. The child will be well and non-toxic. Examination will reveal a limitation of abduction with the hip flexed. Otherwise all will be normal.

A X-ray of the hip will reveal combinations of the classical features. These include cyst formation in the subcapital region together with flattening, fragmentation, and condenstion of the epiphyseal region. Some of these changes can be subtle in the early stages of the disease. Children with proven or suspected Perthes' disease should be referred to an orthopedic surgeon who can consider further management.

Bilateral Perthes' disease is rare (<5% of patients). If bilateral asymmetrical epiphyses are present, spondyloepiphyseal dysplasia or hypothyroidism should be considered.

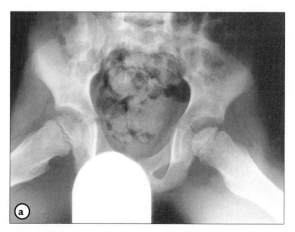

Figure 5.3 a

Frog leg view of the hips. This demonstrates a subchondral fissure and increased density of the left proximal femoral epiphysis. The changes are typical of early Perthes' disease.

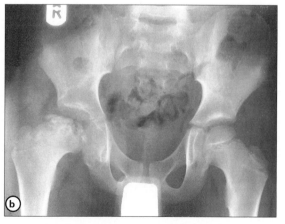

Figure 5.3 b

Anteroposterior view of the hips. This demonstrates long-standing Perthes' disease of the right hip. There is condensation, fissure formation, and fragmentation of the right proximal femoral epiphysis together with a modeling defect of the right femoral neck which is expanded—the so-called coxa magna deformity.

SLIPPED UPPER FEMORAL EPIPHYSIS

This is a condition often missed on initial presentation. It commonly affects pre- or peripubertal children. Often there is a history of mild trauma a short while before the onset of symptoms. Symptoms are few but include vague pain in either the hip, knee or both. Knee pain in all children should always lead one to suspect hip pathology. Examination is often normal in the early stages. It is often helpful to observe the child supine on a couch when external rotation of the leg may be seen (**Figure 5.4 a**). In advanced disease, there may be shortening of the leg and painful movements of the hip.

Correct radiology is imperative. A lateral view of the hip is needed in early stages of the disease to show minor slips. Advanced lesions will be visible in all planes. All children with slipped upper femoral epiphysis should be referred to an orthopedic surgeon for further management (**Figure 5.4 b and c**).

THE LIMPING CHILD

This is one of the more common presentations to a pediatric AED. While the possible diagnoses are legion, in practice only a few are common. Apart from the conditions discussed above it is important to exclude malignancy, either primary or secondary, infection, tenosynovitis of the various tendons in the lower limb and occult trauma.

It is essential that a careful history be taken. Trauma should be suspected in the first instance. Active children often sustain trauma not apparent at the time but which shows as a limp after a period of rest. If trauma is suspected, signs of systemic illness will be absent, the child will have a good appetite and will be otherwise well.

Examination of the lower limb should involve observing the gait of the child to confirm the presence of a limp and to ascertain the limb involved. Parents can often be

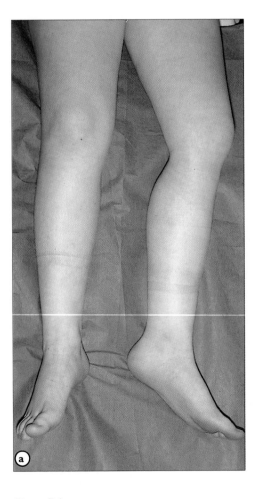

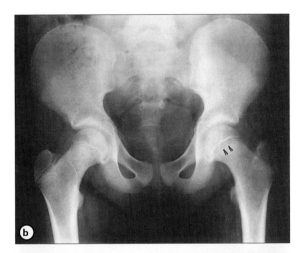

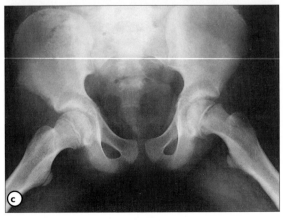

Figure 5.4 a–c

(a) Child with external rotation of the left hip. There is a slip of the left proximal femoral epiphysis, best seen on the lateral film (c). The anterior posterior film (b) shows less obvious abnormality but there is increased translucency and widening of the epiphyseal plate region (arrowheads).

misleading in describing their child's problem! Careful palpation of the limb may reveal focal tenderness. Common areas include the tibia (toddler's fracture) or the foot, either over the calcaneus or the metatarsals. Appropriate X-rays of the foot or calcaneus are needed if foot or heel tenderness is present.

AVASCULAR NECROSIS (Figure 5.6 a–d)

Avascular necrosis can affect many parts of a child's skeleton during different periods of development. One common form is Perthes' disease which has already been discussed.

OSGOOD–SCHLATTER'S DISEASE

Osgood–Schlatter's disease commonly affects peripubertal and adolescent children who are particularly active. They usually present with pain and swelling inferior to the patella over the tibial tuberosity. The child typically is a keen athlete and the affected limb is usually subject to repeated multiple stresses and strains. Occasionally, the area will be hot.

Typical radiographic appearances show fragmentation of the tibial tuberosity with associated soft tissue swelling (**Figure 5.5a and b**).

However, the condition should really be made clinically without recourse to radiology. The child should be advised to avoid all excessive exercise and exercises such as swimming may be encouraged. Usually the pain settles within weeks of cessation of sporting activity and this in itself is usually a good indication of progress of treatment.

Physiotherapy is indicated to maintain muscle bulk in the quadriceps muscle group. Occasionally, the disease is bilateral.

A small number of children require surgery and have painful bone ossicles removed but these are very much in

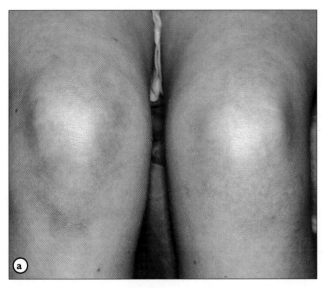

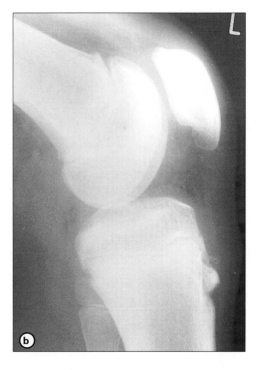

Figure 5.5a and b
(a)Swelling over right tibial tuberosity.
(b)Lateral view of the knee of a child with persistent pain over the proximal tibia. The appearances are typical of Osgood–Schlatter's disease showing soft tissue swelling over the tissue tuberosity. The tuberosity itself is irregular.

the minority. Other areas affected by avascular necrosis are detailed in the table below.

KNEE PAIN IN CHILDREN

Children, particularly girls, often present with knee pain. The history is usually vague but occasionally a good history of injury is obtained. In this situation one should avidly look for ligamentous or epiphyseal injury. The presence of a loose body should also be suspected.

In most cases, no defining moment of trauma is found. Radiographs of the knee should be taken. Usually these are normal, but occasionally evidence of osteochondritis dissecans is seen. This should be referred to an orthopedic surgeon as the loose fragment may be surgically replaced.

Retropatellar pain is common. On examination, compression of the patella against the femoral condyles may elicit pain. Plain radiology may occasionally show abnor-

malities and should be performed at least once to rule out significant pathology.

In most cases, there is little emergency treatment to be offered except physiotherapy to maintain quadriceps bulk, and gentle exercises. Otherwise the child should be referred to an orthopedic surgeon for further assessment.

PULLED ELBOW

Pulled elbow (or nursemaid's elbow as it is sometimes known) is a common reason for children to present. It is often under diagnosed and over-investigated.

Typically, the child is in the younger age group (1 to 4 years old) and presents with a history of not using one of his or her arms (*see* opposite, **Figure 5.7 a**). Further questioning will elicit a history of traction in approximately 70% of cases. This may take the form of the child being pulled along, lifted by the arm or being swung around in play. **If this clinical picture is not present one must exclude any other significant pathology.**

In a minority of cases (<10%) a history of a fall will be present. In the remainder, no history of injury will be available. These children should have a full examination and usually an X-ray, before any further treatment is offered, to exclude pathology such as supracondylar fracture or other injury to the upper or lower arm.

At this stage the child and family need to be handled with care. If a good history of traction is obtained it is possible to gently manipulate the elbow as follows. The affected arm should be held in the doctor's contralateral arm, i.e. a pulled right elbow is held in the doctor's left hand. The doctor then moves to shake the child's hand with his or her free hand (**Figure 5.7 b**). The affected elbow

---

Avascular necrosis in children

Metatarsal head	Freiberg's disease
Navicular bone	Kohler's disease
Heel/Calcaneum	Sever's disease
Tibial tuberocity	Osgood-Schlatter's disease
Proximal femoral epiphysis	Perthes disease
Vertebral bodies	Scheuermann's disease
Capitellum	Panner's disease
Lunate	Keinbock's disease

Figure 5.6 a

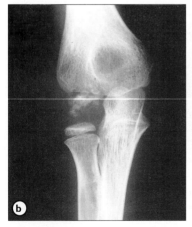

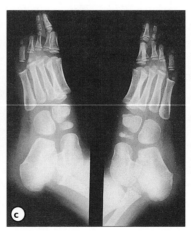

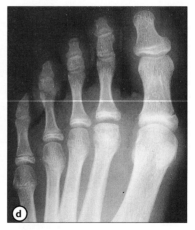

Figure 5.6 b Anterior Posterior view of the right elbow. This demonstrates fragmentation and increased density of the capitellum. The appearances are typical of osteochondritis or Panners' disease.

Figure 5.6 c
Oblique view of both feet. The patient complained of pain in the right tarsal area. There is fragmentation and fissure formation in the right navicular bone. The appearances are of Kohler's disease.

Figure 5.6 d
Radiograph of the right forefoot showing flattening and increased density of the head of the 2nd metatarsal. The appearances are of Kohler–Freiberg's disease.

is then taken gently into the first hand and the elbow gently moved into 90° of flexion. Using the thumb over the radial head, and the hand around the elbow, the doctor's two hands are compressed and the child's wrist pronated. Usually there will be a palpable click, occasionally audible to all. The child will scream but will settle quickly. Failure to feel a click will lead to manipulation as above but this time the forearm will be **supinated** until a click is heard or felt.

Once successful, the child should be allowed to wait in the waiting area for a few minutes during which time normal function can be seen to return. An explanation to the parents of the lesion and how to prevent recurrence can be given. Usually the perpetrator is very embarrassed and will be extremely relieved that he or she has not broken the child's arm!

Failure to feel a click on a second attempt means:
- The diagnosis is wrong
- The technique is wrong

In this situation a more senior colleague should be called.

Often a senior colleague will successfully manipulate the elbow. Occasionally, both will fail. In this situation the child should be placed in a collar and cuff support and allowed home. The child should be reviewed in a day or two when, often, all has settled. Failure to settle at this stage should lead one to treat this as a fracture to an epiphysis around the elbow.

OVERUSE INJURY

Tenosynovitis is an inflammation of the tendon sheath associated with excessive use of the area. Common areas for this to occur are the wrist joint (de Quervain's tenosynovitis), peroneal tendons, Achilles tendon, hamstrings and groin. Typically, the child will present reporting pain around the affected tendon of 2–3 days' duration. A history of overuse up to a week before the onset of pain may be obtained. If one traces back this far a cause will usually be identified. Children with tendon pain around the ankle and foot are usually very active and participate in sports such as dancing, ballet, and judo.

It is important to assess the activity that the child undertakes together with the way that they participate. Footwear should be assessed for foot and leg problems.

Once a diagnosis of tendon injury has been made the child should be referred to physiotherapy as soon as possible. The physiotherapist, who should be familiar with pediatric sports or overuse injury, should start treatment aimed at resolving the acute problem . Additionally, advice should be given on the correct way to participate in the sport in question and also on the most suitable footwear and other aids to use.

Occasionally, a short course of a non-steroidal anti-inflammatory drug (NSAID) is required. Ibuprofen, 20 mg/kg/day in divided doses, will usually be effective within 3–4 days. If there has been no change in symptoms on this dosage there is no point in continuing with NSAIDs. Most children's symptoms will be resolved when using such regimes and only a few will require steroid injections. This treatment is outside the remit of an AED and should really be undertaken by a rheumatologist.

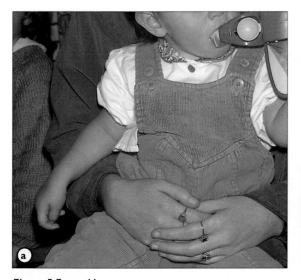
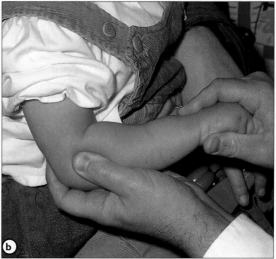

Figure 5.7 a and b
(a) Typical appearance of a child with right 'pulled elbow'. (b) Position of the operator's hands prior to manipulation.

BACK PAIN

Back pain is extremely rare in childhood and when present should not be ignored. Two diagnoses will be discussed:

- Discitis.
- Spondylolisthesis.

DISCITIS

Discitis is an infective lesion of the intravertebral disks. The causal pathogen is typically *S. aureus*. The infection is usually low grade and manifests itself as non-specific back pain. Occasionally, pain can be present in the abdomen, particularly in the inguinal region. Blood cultures will typically be negative but there will be a raised ESR. Magnetic resonance imaging is extremely helpful (**Figure 5.8**). If diagnosed, the child should be referred to an orthopedic surgeon for further management.

SPONDYLOLISTHESIS

This condition can either be congenital or traumatic. Congenital lesions are associated with other spinal abnormalities and are extremely rare. Of more concern is the peri-adolescent child who begins to complain of low-back pain. Typically, it is an active boy participating in contact sports such as rugby or football. The pain is due to stress fractures in either or both pars interarticularis of the lumbar vertebrae. This usually involves the L5/S1 area. The pain is intermittent in nature but can be quite severe. Anteroposterior, lateral, and oblique X-rays of the spine can often confirm the diagnosis. Isotope bone scanning will show an the area of increased activity (**Figure 5.9 a–c**).

Fracture and complete separation of both pars interarticularis will result in complete spondylolisthesis which may require surgery. Most cases, however, can be managed conservatively but an orthopedic opinion, particularly from someone with an interest in sports injuries, is advised.

Other causes of back pain in children should also be considered. These will include neoplastic infiltration of the cord, vertebrae, or both, and osteomyelitis . **Back pain in children is seldom mechanical, as in the older population, and osteopathic manipulation should not be carried out until all the possible underlying causes have been excluded.**

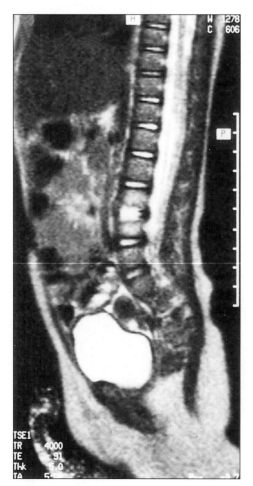

Figure 5.8
Sagittal T2-weighted MR image of the lumbar spine. This demonstrates a high signal within the L3/L4 intervertebral disk space. The disk space is expanded. There is a small posterior protrusion into the spinal canal. The increased signal is also seen in the adjacent vertebral bodies.

ACUTE TORTICOLLIS

It is not infrequent for children to present to the department with spontaneous onset of pain in the neck. Occasionally, the precipitating episode will be obvious; for example, the child says that he or she turned round suddenly and felt immediate pain. More often than not there will be no such history with the child waking up with the problem (**Figure 5.10**).

It is important to exclude a history of trauma, particularly flexion or compression injury (*see* Trauma: Chapter 4). A history of sore throat or respiratory infection should be sought. On clinical examination, all movements of the cervical spine will be restricted by pain and spasm in the muscles around the neck. The trapezius muscle is often involved. One should look for underlying causes such as tender glands.

There is no indication to X-ray these children unless trauma or other pathology is suspected. If respiratory infection or tonsillitis is suspected, a throat swab can be sent to virology and bacteriology for analysis.

The child should be given analgesia (*see* above), a collar and be referred to physiotherapy. The child should be reviewed in 24–48 hours to ensure movement is returning.

Any other presentation should be viewed with caution. Painless torticollis or gradual onset of torticollis are warning signs of a more significant underlying pathology. In these situations neoplasia, spinal cord lesions or neurologic problems should be considered.

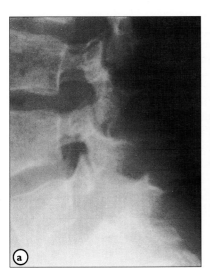
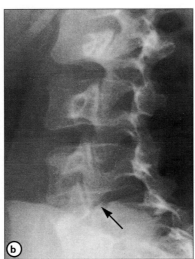
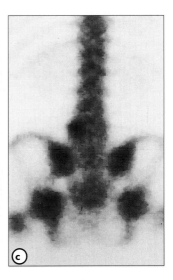

Figure 5.9a–c
(a) Lateral and (b) oblique views of the lumbosacral junction in a child with chronic back pain. Lateral X-rays demonstrate an oblique defect through the pars interarticularis. This was confirmed with the oblique film which shows a 'collar on the dog' (arrowed). (c) Tc99 Methylene diphosphonate bone scan in a child with chronic back pain. This shows an area of increased activity to the left of the midline at the L4 level. Radiographs subsequently revealed a spondylolysis defect.

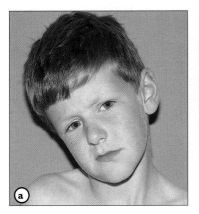
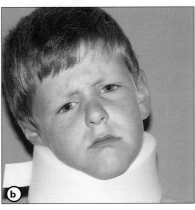

Figure 5.10 a and b
Acute torticollis. (a) This child presented with acute spasm in his neck. Note the marked deviation to one side. (b) This is only partially corrected by the application of a cervical collar. It is more important to administer NSAIDs and to give early active physiotherapy. Unless underlying disease is present, the condition should resolve within 24–48 hours.

CYSTIC SWELLINGS
BAKER'S CYST
A Baker's cyst is an enlargement of the popliteal bursae. It can be quite dramatic and worrying for parents. Typically, it will be slightly fluctuant, but will disappear on flexing the knee. Occasionally, in older children, it can rupture into the calf giving severe pain (**Figure 5.11**).

GANGLION (Figure 5.12)
A ganglion is a herniation of the synovium of a tendon sheath. It can be quite tense and hard. Their sudden appearance often causes parents to worry. Transillumination can help confirm the diagnosis. If there is parental concern the child should be referred to an orthopedic surgeon. Otherwise, a waiting approach can be taken.

ABDOMINAL PAIN

Abdominal pain is a common problem in childhood. While the possible differential diagnosis is wide, in practice, only a small number of diagnoses need to be seriously considered in the first instance. The purpose of this section is to highlight common conditions and to give some indication as to their management in the accident and emergency setting.

ACUTE APPENDICITIS
This is one of the more common surgical emergencies. Typically, the child will present with pain of variable duration. In young children and infants the classical history of central abdominal pain gradually settling in the right iliac fossa is rarely obtained. This typical presentation should be sought in older children. Anorexia, malaise, and fever are other clues of appendicitis.

Examination in the early stages can be both difficult and unreliable. As the inflammation in the appendix increases the signs of guarding and rebound tenderness localize to the right iliac fossa.

Investigations to help the diagnosis include urinalysis, full blood count and, possibly, ultrasound scanning of the appendix area (**Figure 5.13**). However, none are absolutely reliable and good clinical examination is mandatory.

If the diagnosis is suspected, the child should be referred to a surgical team for further assessment.

PERFORATED APPENDIX
If acute appendicitis is allowed to progress the organ will perforate, discharging pus and fecal matter into the peritoneal cavity. The child will rapidly become toxic with signs of peritonitis present. Immediate management in the Accident and Emergency room will involve rapid resuscitation along standard principles. The child should receive 20 ml/kg of normal saline as a rapid bolus. Blood should be sent for a full blood count and blood cultures. Antibiotics should be given early, according to local sensitivities, to be effective against coliforms and anaerobes. Analgesia should not be withheld but given as described in Chapter 4. The child should be referred to the surgical team as soon as possible.

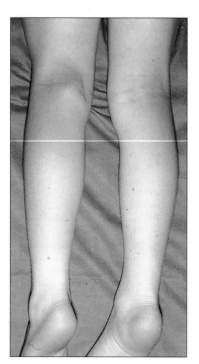

Figure 5.11
Baker's cyst. This is a painless swelling in the popliteal bursa. Usually, it is asymptomatic. This child has a swelling in the left popliteal fossa which disappears when the knee is flexed. Occasionally, Baker's cysts can give rise to pain in the calf when they rupture.

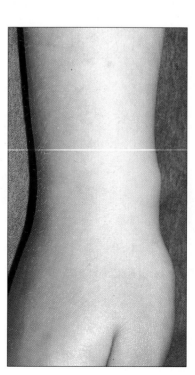

Figure 5.12
Ganglion. This child presented with sudden onset of pain and swelling over the radial aspect of his wrist. This is a ganglion of flexor carpi radialis.

INTUSSUSCEPTION

This a condition affecting boys more than girls and more common in the first year of life. The classically taught triad of abdominal mass, bloody stool, and abdominal pain is frequently absent making this a difficult condition to diagnose.

Intussusception may follow a viral illness, gastroenteritis or Henoch–Schönlein purpura; in most cases no predisposing illness is present.

Many will present collapsed and in need of resuscitation. Here the diagnosis can be difficult to make. Often the work-up will be similar to that of a septic child, including a lumbar puncture, the diagnosis only being considered after sepsis has been ruled out, or symptoms and signs of intussusception become apparent.

The pain of intussusception is colicky and intermittent. The parents may describe the infant as drawing his or her knees into the abdomen, screaming and then going quiet. Examination may reveal a sausage-shaped mass in the abdomen. The stool, described as being like redcurrant jelly, may contain blood, either fresh or altered.

If suspected of suffering from an intussusception, the child should undergo standard resuscitation as appropriate. Blood should be taken for a full blood count and urea and electrolytes and also sent for 'group and save'. A plain X-ray of the abdomen may show abnormalities in the area of the intussusception (*see* **Figure 5.14,**). The presence of dilated loops of gut suggests obstruction. Analgesia in the form of intravenous opiates will help make the child more comfortable.

An ultrasound scan is helpful in the diagnosis (*see* **Figure 5.15**). Once diagnosed, the child should be referred to the receiving surgeons who will consider the options of hydrostatic reduction and operative reduction (*see* **Figure 5.16**).

URINARY TRACT INFECTION

Abdominal pain and nausea or vomiting are common and non-specific symptoms presenting to the emergency room. Urinary tract infection should be excluded as these symptoms are often the only symptoms present as the cause. Further management is discussed in Chapter 3.

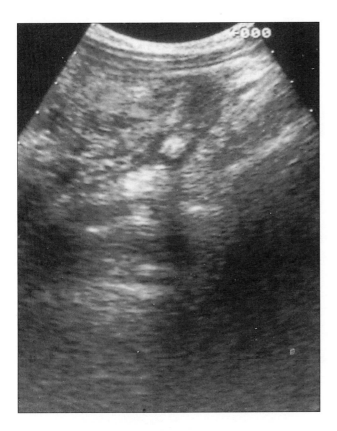

Figure 5.13
Ultrasound examination of the abnormal appendix. This reveals a dilated appendix containing appendicolith.

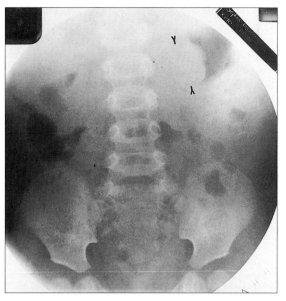

Figure 5.14
Plain film of the abdomen in a child with intussusception. The soft tissue density of the intussuscepting mass is outlined by arrows in the transverse colon.

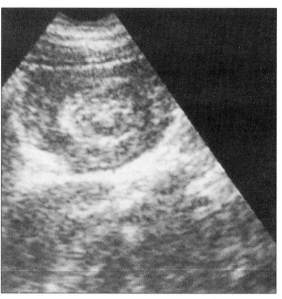

Figure 5.15
Ultrasound section through the intussusception showing a typical target appearance.

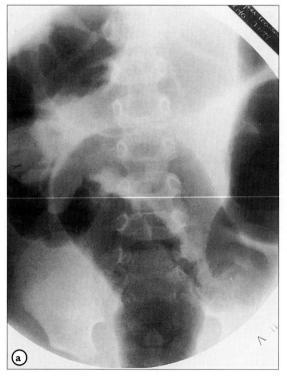

Figure 5.16 a
(a) Air reduction of the intussusception. Arrows indicate the intussusception, now in the cecum.

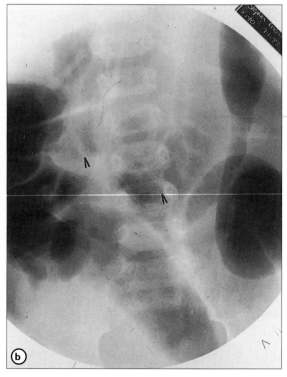

Figure 5.16 b
(b) Total reduction of the intussusception. The mass has now disappeared and there is free-filling of the small bowel with gas (arrows).

HEPATITIS A

Hepatitis is a common cause of abdominal pain, nausea and vomiting in childhood. It tends to occur sporadically in epidemics with some children presenting with more acute problems than others. Typically presentation will be one of viral illness with non-descript features of fever, malaise and nausea. These may precede the development of jaundice. The jaundice may be subtle and mild, being diagnosed only on laboratory testing (anicteric hepatitis).

Simple tests that may help confirm the diagnosis will be a rise in the levels of urobilinogen and bilirubin in the urine.

Hepatitis A, is usually a mild disease in childhood and the child can safely be allowed home. The parents should be advised about hygiene and the possible transmission to siblings or friends.

MEDICAL CAUSES OF ABDOMINAL PAIN

Pneumonia and diabetic ketoacidosis can both present with abdominal pain. This only emphasizes the need for all children to have a full examination including chest examination and urinalysis.

Migraine can present as severe abdominal pain. It is associated with a family history of migraine. The child may also have classical migraine, with headache, vomiting or fortification spectra accompanying the abdominal pain. Pizotifen may be useful in both terminating the attack or as prophylaxis.

This is often a diagnosis of exclusion and other causes of abdominal pain need to be excluded before the diagnosis is entertained.

RECURRENT ABDOMINAL PAIN IN CHILDHOOD

Many children present with long-standing abdominal pain of vague origin and uncertain etiology. Many will have been seen repeatedly by the family practitioner and may have already been admitted for observation. There will often be a considerable degree of parental anxiety (quite understandably) which can make the situation difficult for junior doctors.

In these circumstances it is incumbent on junior doctors to avoid dismissing these children out of hand. A full history and examination must be performed and the urine tested. The aim is to exclude all the above diagnoses with a minimum of investigation. A normal ultrasound examination can be a useful adjunct to allay parents and doctors anxiety. It is usually negative. If all is normal and the abdomen is quiescent to physical examination, it is probably safe to allow the child home to be followed-up either by the family practitioner or in the surgical outpatients department. If allowed home, parents should be counseled as to further management if symptoms in keeping with more serious pathology occur. In the event of the doctor being unable to reassure himself that the abdomen is quiescent, a surgical opinion should be obtained with a view to admitting the child for further observation and/or investigation. Even if no pathology is found and the child is discharged after only a few hours, it is often reassuring to the parents.

INGUINAL HERNIAE

These are more common in males than females. While they can occur at any age they are most common in early childhood. Premature infants are more prone to herniae than full-term babies (**Figure 5.17**).

Typically, there will be a variable abdominal swelling present in the lower abdomen. Swelling will be increased by intra-abdominal pressure brought on by crying or straining. Often no swelling will be seen when the doctor examines the child but the history is so clearcut that there

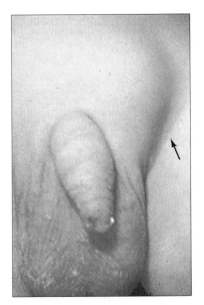

Figure 5.17
This child has an inguinal hernia which is most prominent when the child is crying. This should be referred for surgical opinion.

should be no doubt as to the diagnosis. If further confirmation is required, stimulating the child to induce crying may produce the swelling. Once diagnosed, the child should be referred for a surgical opinion.

A persistent swelling that does not disappear suggests that the bowel within is incarcerated. If left untreated this will progress to strangulation. This should be referred urgently for a surgical opinion.

SCROTAL SWELLINGS

HYDROCELES (Figure 5.18)

Hydroceles are due to persistence of the processus vaginalis. The potential space is filled with fluid that can be readily transilluminated. They may require surgical intervention, particularly if there is an associated hernia. For this reason a referral to a pediatric surgeon should be made.

TESTICULAR TORSION

Testicular torsion is a surgical emergency which is often underdiagnosed. The onset of pain in the testicle in young boys should lead one to suspect this diagnosis as opposed to epididymitis (**Figure 5.19**).

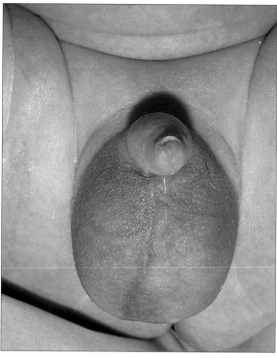

Figure 5.18
Hydrocele. This child presented with painless swelling in the left side of his scrotum. It was noticed by his mother when she was bathing him. The painless nature of the swelling, transillumination and the clinical picture suggested that a hydrocele was present. This was confirmed on ultrasound.

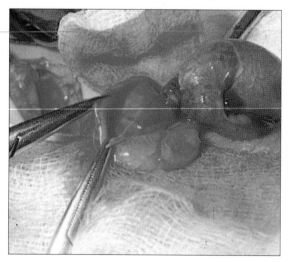

Figure 5.19
Testicular torsion. This gangrenous testicle was exposed at operation. The child had pain in the left testicle for 12 hours prior to presentation.

All boys with testicular pain should be referred as an emergency to a surgeon who will consider the differential diagnosis and probably consider exploration of the testicle.

IDIOPATHIC SCROTAL EDEMA

Idiopathic scrotal edema is a disease of unknown etiology. Typically, there will be redness and swelling of the scrotum; this will often be unilateral. It may extend down to the adjoining thigh and groin. It is self-limiting and requires no active treatment. Having said this, testicular torsion must be excluded (**Figure 5.20**).

ASPIRATED FOREIGN BODY

It is not unusual for children to aspirate coins or other large objects. Often they wedge in the esophagus at the level of the cricoid and cause considerable distress. It is difficult at times to distinguish between these foreign bodies in the esophagus from those in the airway. Often drooling will be present and the child may be unable to speak due to the discomfort in the area of the larynx.

If a foreign body in the esophagus is suspected, the child should go to the X-ray department escorted by a senior member of the medical staff. Lateral views of the neck should be taken to confirm the position of the foreign body (**Figure 5.21**). If the foreign body is radiolucent, further radiographic techniques may be required, such as a water soluble contrast swallow. Once the presence of a foreign body is confirmed, radiographic removal should be considered .

RADIOGRAPHIC REMOVAL OF A FOREIGN BODY

The child is brought to the screening room and mildly sedated. The child is then placed in the lateral position on the screening table. A Foley catheter is passed down the esophagus past the foreign body. The balloon is filled with radiopaque solution and the Foley catheter is gently withdrawn back through the esophagus. The balloon impacts on the foreign body and the foreign body can usually be loosened with gentle upper traction (**Figure 5.22**). Once in the mouth the foreign body can be removed with forceps. Most children tolerate this procedure well and the failure rate is very low.

If the foreign body is firmly impacted or is found to be well down the esophagus, i.e. beyond the length of the Foley catheter, removal via an endoscope may be indicated.

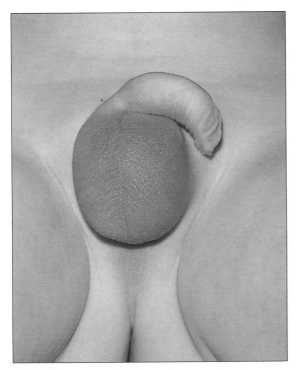

Figure 5.20
Idiopathic scrotal edema. This child presented with spontaneous onset of a red, edematous scrotum and base of penis. Occasionally, this can spread onto the thighs and perineum. Differential diagnosis should include testicular torsion and infection.

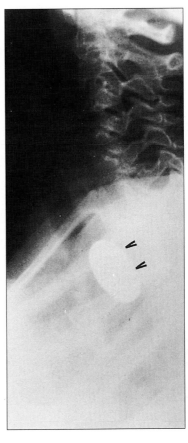

Figure 5.21
Plain film showing a child with a coin lodged in the esophagus at the level of the aortic arch (arrowheads).

INTRA-ABDOMINAL FOREIGN BODIES

It is not uncommon for children to put things in their mouth and either deliberately or accidentally swallow them. Of prime importance is to exclude the foreign body in the airway. It is usual for the foreign body to pass through the esophagus and will be somewhere in the gastrointestinal tract. The position will depend upon the timing of ingestion and the time the child presents (**Figure 5.23**).

Most foreign bodies are found in the stomach and can be safely left to pass through. The one exception to this is button batteries. These can cause significant problems no matter where they lodge. Two potential problems exist:

1. Fresh batteries can erode through mucosal membranes. In the gastrointestinal tract this can lead to viscus perforation.
2. Older batteries can disintegrate and if they contain mercuric salts, toxic levels of mercury can be released.

Great care, therefore, must be taken in the management of button batteries. If the battery is in the upper gastrointestinal tract it must be removed as a matter of urgency, either via endoscope or magnetic retrieval, under X-ray control.

If the battery has passed further into the gastrointestinal tract a decision must be made as to whether laparotomy is warranted especially if the battery is suspected of being lodged or whether it is safe to watch its passage through the bowel.

FOREIGN BODY ELSEWHERE

A foreign body in the nose or ear is a common reason for children to present to the AED. Often the object will have been present for some time, only becoming apparent when a foul smelling discharge supervenes. These foreign bodies can be difficult to remove. (**Figure 5.24**)

The ease of removal of foreign bodies depends on the cooperation of the child, the nature of the object, the duration of impaction, and the skill of the operator. One or two attempts only should be made by the first clinician to see the child. After that, the child will be less cooperative and specialist help should be sought.

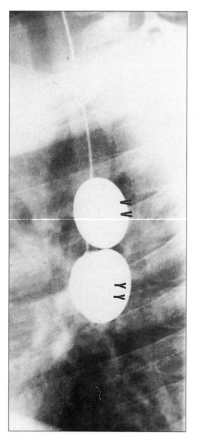

Figure 5.22
Removal of a coin using a Foley catheter (arrows indicate contrast in the Foley balloon; arrowheads the coin in the esophagus).

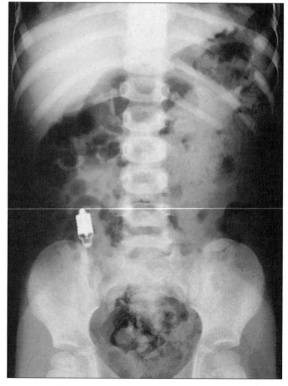

Figure 5.23
Plain abdominal X-ray showing an ingested torch bulb lying in the cecum.

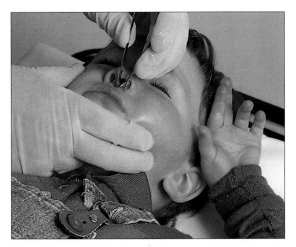

Figure 5.24
Removal of a foreign body from the left nostril of a cooperative child.

SOFT TISSUE INFECTIONS

Infections are a relatively frequent reason for children to present to the AED. Often, treatment will have been started by the family doctor and they will be referred for management of non-resolving or worsening lesions.

Types of skin and soft tissue infection in children include:
* Bacterial infections.
* Viral infections.
* Fungal infections.

BACTERIAL INFECTIONS

Bacterial infections are by far the most common reason for children to present. Typically, they present with either a cellulitis or abscess formation.

The most common organism found is *S. aureus* but Streptococcal infection is also common. Enteric organisms should be expected around the perineum and buttocks.

The reason behind the development of skin infections is unclear. Clearly, there has been a breach of the normal barrier presented by the skin to infection. Often this will be minor unrecognized trauma, but the possibility of occult penetrating trauma will also have to be considered. This history will seldom be obtained in young children.

Commonly, in infections around the hands and face, there is a history of nail biting and poor hygiene.

Typical antibiotic regimes which **might** be used for the treatment of soft tissue infections appear in **Figure 5.25**.

GENERAL PRINCIPLES

Children with skin infections fall into two categories: toxic or non-toxic. Toxic children will have evidence of septicemia suggested by tachycardia, tachypnea and elevated temperature with or without systemic collapse. Most infections, however, do not have any systemic involvement. Toxic children should be admitted for intravenous therapy while most of the non-toxic children will be eligible for treatment at home with close outpatient follow-up. Occasionally, non-toxic children will have to be admitted for incision and drainage of an abcess, and intravenous antibiotics. In these situations the child will have to be kept fasted and it is sensible to commence intravenous therapy with a view to converting to oral antibiotics as soon as possible after the anesthetic.

In general, pus should be drained surgically using adequate and appropriate anesthesia. Often this will require a general anesthetic as children may not tolerate local anesthesia. Also it will not be possible to achieve local block with many abscesses. Ethyl chloride use is mentioned only to be condemned.

It is wise to check the urine or blood sugar in all children with skin infection. While it is a rare presentation of diabetes it would be unfortunate to miss it.

TREATMENT
Poultices
Many clinicians use magnesium sulphate as a poultice. Many herbalists will apply potions such as cold porridge, tea and bread, and various other compounds to the affected area in an effort to draw pus. There is no evidence that they do so. However, applying a poultice may have the following benefits:
* A lotion is applied to the area and this may have psychological benefits.
* The poultice will have to be applied with some form of retaining dressing on top thereby preventing the child (or parent) from poking or interfering with the infection.
* It may actually provide some degree of splintage to the local area.
* Many poultices are soothing to the inflamed area.

All of these are good reasons for applying a poultice and we do not discourage the practice.

Antibiotic therapy for soft tissue infections		
Organism		**Antibiotic**
	First-line	*Second-line (if penicillin allergy)*
Staphylococcus aureus	flucloxacillin	erythromycin
Streptococcus	penicillin	erythromycin
Anaerobic organisms	metronidazole	co-trimoxazole
Enteric organisms	co-amoxiclav	cephalosporin

Figure 5.25

HAND INFECTIONS

Paronychiae, pulp space infections and web space infections are all seen frequently within the AED setting.

Paronychia (Figure 5.26)

These usually present either as cellulitis around the nail or with frank pus present. Cellulitis should be treated with oral antibiotics e.g. flucloxacillin or erythromycin and early review at 24 hours should be arranged. Frank pus should be drained and mupirocin cream applied to the surface. The child should be started on antibiotics and reviewed at 2 or 3 days. Occasionally, pus will have developed under the nail and the nail may have to be removed to obtain complete drainage.

Frequent or recurrent paronychia may be associated with a carrier state of Staphylococcus. Swabs of the nose and axillae may grow Staphylococci, suggesting further treatment. Parents should also be considered as carriers.

Pulp space infection (Figure 5.27)

These are extremely painful. Often the children present in the early hours of the morning. First-line treatment

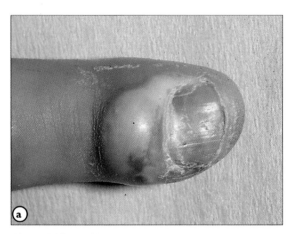 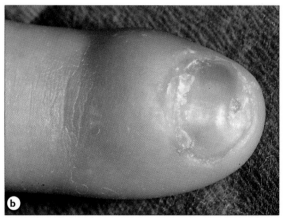

Figure 5.26 a and b
Paronychia. Paronychia is very common in childhood particularly when nail hygiene is poor. (a) This will probably only require simple incision and drainage. (b) Shows subungual infection. This will almost certainly require the nail to be avulsed for this to be drained properly.

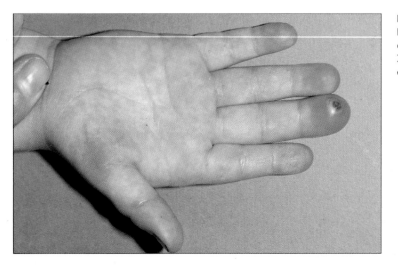

Figure 5.27
Pulp space infection which was allowed to develop to suppuration. This will require an X-ray prior to incision and drainage to exclude underlying osteomyelitis.

should be with antibiotics (flucloxacillin or erythromycin) but the child should be reviewed early. Pulp-space infections will often suppurate and the pus will need to be drained. The infection is usually deeper than is apparent on initial examination. If allowed to progress, necrosis may occur in the nail tuft with resultant osteomyelitis setting in.

Web space infection (Figure 5.28)

These infections are deeper than is apparent on initial examination. It is tempting to drain the blister with small amounts of pus being expressed. This will only lead to further worsening of the situation as the abscess develops in the web space. These should be drained properly under general anesthetic.

PERI-ORBITAL CELLULITIS (Figure 5.29)

This is a serious and significant infection in children. It carries a risk of significant morbidity associated with cavernous sinus thrombosis. All children with peri-orbital cellulitis should be admitted for intravenous antibiotics. These are occasionally associated with underlying sinusitis caused

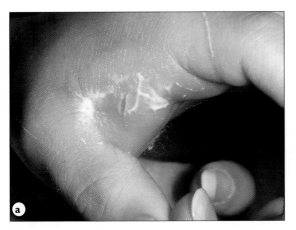

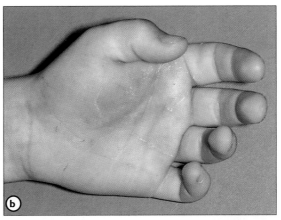

Figure 5.28 a and b
Web space infection. (a) Superficial infection in the web space. (b) Extension into the palm. The hand has been held in a position of

function as all movements of the fingers are painful. This can spread further into the wrist into the space of Parona. This requires excision and drainage under general anesthetic.

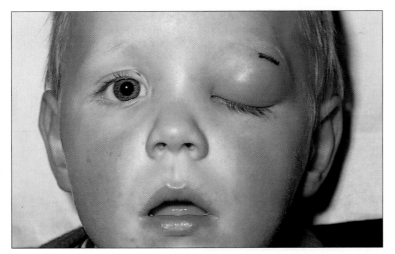

Figure 5.29
Peri-orbital cellulitis, secondary to a wound in the eyebrow region.

by Streptococci or *H. influenzae*; Staphylococci have also been implicated. For this reason initial treatment should be with intravenous flucloxacillin and ampicillin.

CONJUNCTIVITIS (Figure 5.30)

- Bacterial.
- Viral.
- Allergic.
- Trauma-related.

The differences between these can be very difficult to determine clinically. As a general rule, single eye involvement is usually due to bacterial infection. Inflammation affecting both eyes, or other mucous membranes, will usually be due to viral or allergic causes.

Bacterial conjunctivitis is usually caused by *H. influenzae* or *S. aureus*. Typically, the eye is red and injected. If old enough the child may complain of a gritty feeling under the eyelid. Before treatment, an attempt should be made to document eye function and visual acuity. Treatment with antibiotic ointment or drops should be started only when eye swabs have been taken. Most organisms are sensitive to chloramphenicol eye preparations but sodium fusidate may also be used. The child should be reviewed early with the swab results and treatment changed according to progress and reported sensitivities. Any failure to progress should be referred to an ophthalmologist. Chlamydial infection may be slow to resolve with the above treatment. Specific techniques are needed to culture chlamydia. This should be discussed with the local bacteriology specialists.

Viral conjunctivitis may be associated with other viral illness or occur alone (**Figure 5.31**). As discussed, it may be difficult to diagnose and distinguish from other causes. One particular form must be recognized however. This is a dendritic ulcer caused by herpes simplex virus infection.

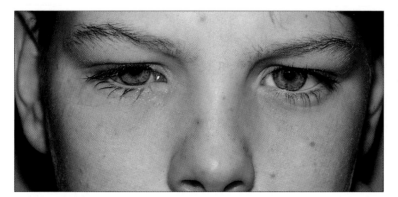

Figure 5.30
This young man has an acutely inflamed right eye. Unilateral bacterial conjunctivitis was suspected. *Haemophilus influenzae* was cultured from a swab taken prior to treatment with chloramphenicol.

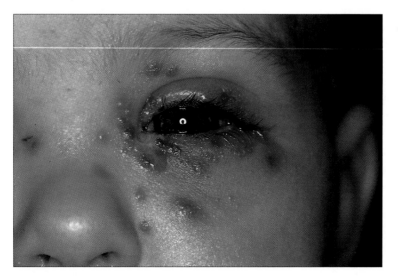

Figure 5.31
Vesicular lesion in the left peri-orbital region. Viral swabs confirmed these as herpes simplex. There is no eye involvement yet.

The characteristic branching chains are pathognomonic of this condition.

Allergic conjunctivitis will occur whenever the child is exposed to an allergen to which he is sensitive. It is usually associated with rhinitis. Sodium cromoglycate drops and antihistamines may give added relief.

Other causes of acute red eye are rare in childhood but must be considered. An indication that they are present may be gleaned from physical examination, ophthalmoscopy or by failure to respond to simple treatment. A fuller discussion of eye pathology is beyond the remit of this book.

IMPETIGO

This can be either staphylococcal or streptococcal in origin. Treatment should be with antibiotics, both systemically and topically. We recommend mupirocin topically together with either flucloxacillin or penicillin depending on the organism involved.

OTITIS MEDIA

Otitis media is one of the most common ailments in childhood with most cases occurring before the age of five. The etiology of the condition may be viral, bacterial or bacterial superimposed on viral. Classically, the child presents with fever, pain and general malaise. The pain can be quite severe and may require considerable analgesia. Common organisms causing otitis media are:

- *H. influenzae*.
- *Streptococcus pneumoniae*.
- *Moraxella catarrhalis* (formerly *Branhamella catarrhalis*).
- Virus.

It can be difficult to determine viral from bacterial causes but some general rules apply. Viral illness will affect more than one mucous membrane and be associated with other symptoms such as coryza, rash or conjunctivitis. Bacterial infection will usually be unilateral and may often be associated with a preceding viral illness.

Treatment is symptomatic with analgesia in adequate doses, antipyretics, if indicated, and antibiotics for bacterial cases. The role of antibiotics is questioned in some quarters. Antibiotics are indicated if systemic signs (e.g. pyrexia >39°C) are evident. Typically, *S. pneumoniae* or *H. influenzae* are present, therefore antibiotics must be effective against both pathogens. If penicillin-resistant, clarithromycin is the drug of choice.

Complications of otitis media include perforation of the tympanic membrane (**Figure 5.32**), chronic suppurative otitis media, cholesteatoma formation, mastoiditis (**Figure 5.33**) and intracranial infection.

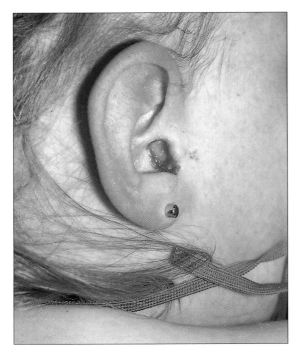

Figure 5.32
Pus draining from the right ear. This is due to suppurtive otitis media and perforation of the tympanic membrane. This child presented with a febrile convulsion.

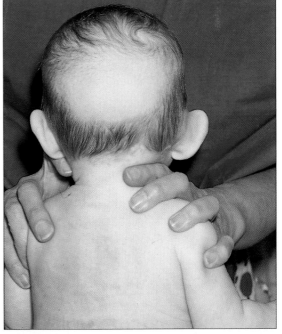

Figure 5.33
Acute mastoiditis. Note the protruding right ear with erythema over the mastoid area.

TONSILLITIS

As with otitis media, tonsillitis is quite common in the under-five age group. Again it may be viral or bacterial. The child may present in pain or with failure to take fluids. Streptococcal infections are often associated with headache and neck stiffness. Again, viral causes will usually have multiple mucous membrane involvement with bacterial causes being more localized. Lymph node enlargement may be present. If particularly tender or swollen, infectious mononucleosis should be suspected—a monospot or Paul–Bunnell test will confirm the diagnosis.

The most common bacteria found in bacterial tonsillitis are Streptococci. Treatment of tonsillitis is by analgesia, antipyretics and antibiotics if throat swab culture reveals streptococci. Penicillin or erythromycin are indicated if streptococcal infection is evident.

CERVICAL GLAND INFECTION (Figure 5.34)

This is a reasonably common presentation in children. Infection in the lymph glands of the neck, followed by suppuration within the gland, is often associated with severe upper respiratory tract infection. These glands are often tender but the child is usually systemically well. Associated organisms include Streptococci, Staphylococci and *H. influenzae*. Most will resolve with oral antibiotics, but as surgical intervention is often indicated, early follow-up in surgical outpatients is recommended. Ultrasound can help determine swollen glands from pus.

CELLULITIS (Figure 5.35)

Cellulitis is more common in the limbs but again can appear anywhere. Typically, there will be erythema associated with increased temperature and pain on palpation. Usually the child is systemically well and treatment with oral antibiotics is adequate. If the child is toxic, admission for intravenous therapy is indicated. Usually the infection is caused by Streptococci but Staphylococci can also be implicated.

ASCENDING LYMPHANGITIS (Figure 5.36)

This is a variant on cellulitis with streptococcal infection affecting the lymph vessels. Typically, there will be a red, erythematous line extending proximally from an innocuous lesion in the limb. If toxic, the child should be admitted for intravenous antibiotics. Otherwise, outpatient therapy is indicated with next day follow-up. Failure to resolve quickly should lead to the child being admitted for intravenous therapy.

ABSCESS (Figure 5.37)

Abscesses are usually associated with staphylococcal infection although other organisms are also implicated. There are several stages in the development of an abscess:

- Erythema and hardening.
- Suppuration.
- Discharge.

If caught in the early stages, oral antibiotics may be adequate. Most, however, progress relentlessly to suppuration and they will either discharge spontaneously or can be assisted to do so by use of the surgeon's knife.

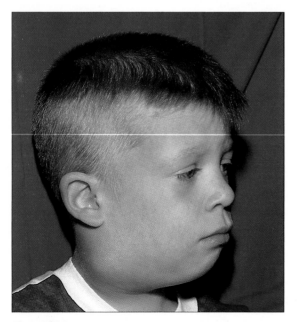

Figure 5.34
Cervical adenitis. This young man has marked swelling in the cervical gland. The differential diagnosis would be that of mumps.

Management

Once suppuration has begun rapid relief will be obtained by draining the pus. Antibiotics are not really indicated at this stage as they will not penetrate into the suppurating material. Some surgeons give a dose of antibiotics prior to incision. The drug is in the serum which penetrates the abscess cavity only after incision.

To drain an abscess one requires adequate analgesia which can only be achieved by general anesthesia. Local anesthetic infiltration is seldom effective.

It is tempting to remove the outer portion of the abscess only, but usually there is a thick layer of inspissated pus located at the bottom of the abscess which needs to be removed, usually by curettage.

There are many ways to deal with the abscess cavity, once it has been drained. These include:
- Packing with gauze or tulle gras, often impregnated with antibiotic or disinfectant.
- Instillation of antibiotic material such as sodium fusidate.
- Early suture of the abscess cavity.

Each of the above, either singly or in combination, have their advocates. There is no absolutely correct way to treat an abscess cavity but probably the most important thing is to drain all the pus, remove all the debris and allow fresh bleeding into the wound to enable the healing process to continue.

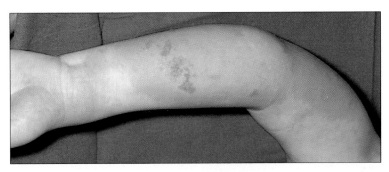

Figure 5.35
Cellulitis. This child has marked cellulitis of the left arm. He was pyrexial and toxic. He was admitted for intravenous antibiotics.

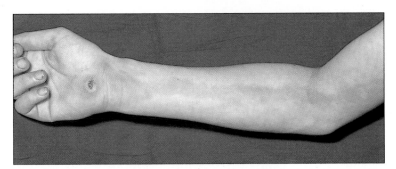

Figure 5.36
Ascending lymphangitis. A minor wound has become infected.

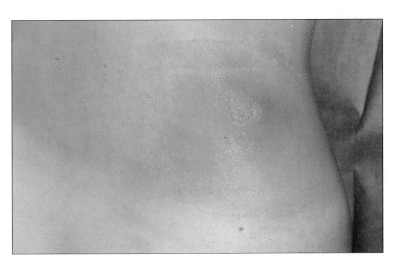

Figure 5.37
An early abscess over the right loin. Note the surrounding erythema and that the abscess is beginning to point.

PYOGENIC GRANULOMA (Figures 5.38 and 5.39)

Pyogenic granuloma is a peculiar entity of unknown etiology. Patients with improperly treated infections, and with wounds that are continually exposed to irritation, are prone to develop this condition.

If present these should be carefully curetted and the tissue sent for histological examination. A tetracycline and cortisone cream should be used and the child reviewed with the results from the histology within one week. **It is important to check histology on these tissues as, occasionally, malignant melanoma can present in this fashion.**

DENTAL ABSCESS AND INFECTION

Dental abscesses need to be referred to a dental surgeon for optimal care of the abscess and teeth (**Figure 5.40**).

PERINEAL AND BUTTOCK INFECTIONS (Figure 5.41)

These can take the form of either cellulitis, abscess or both. Treatment should follow the principles alluded to above for treatment of cellulitis or abscess. One may have to consider anaerobic or enteric organisms as a cause.

Inflammatory bowel disease may also present as abscess or sinus around the anus and perineum.

Buttock and perianal abscesses have the potential to communicate in the form of a fistula with the rectum. For this reason they should be drained by a surgeon in theatre who has the facility to do a sigmoidoscopy or proctoscopy at the time of drainage.

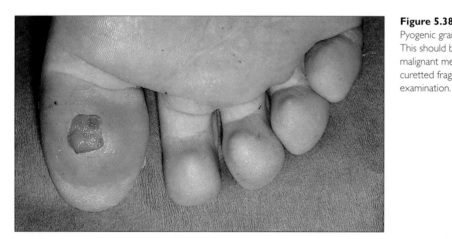

Figure 5.38
Pyogenic granuloma to the sole of the foot. This should be differentiated from a malignant melanoma by sending the curetted fragments for histological examination.

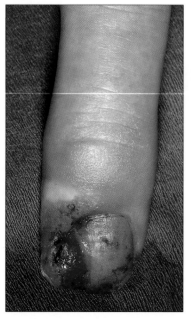

Figure 5.39
An inadequately drained paronychia which has developed into a pyogenic granuloma.

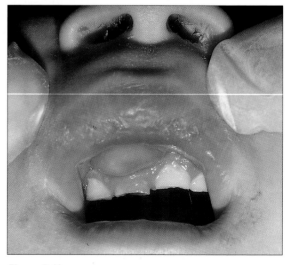

Figure 5.40
Dental abscess. This child has had previous trauma to the upper right incisor which has led to subsequent infection. This should be dealt with by a skilled dental practitioner.

INGROWING TOE NAIL (Figure 5.42)

This condition has many etiologies. Poor foot hygiene, ill-fitting footwear/socks, nail trauma and a familial tendency to ingrowing toe nails have all been implicated.

There is little point in treating these with antibiotics. The underlying pathology is one of a small nail fragment growing in under the skin. The lesion will not resolve until this has been removed. Many procedures exist to ensure that this happens and every operator has his own technique. General anesthesia will usually be required in young children but as they approach adolescence the operation may be done under a local anesthetic. Since many techniques exist it is beyond the scope of this text to explore the subject further.

VIRAL INFECTIONS

Typically, viral infections of the skin present as a painful vesicular lesion. The most common viruses are either herpes simplex or herpes zoster.

HERPES SIMPLEX (Figure 5.43)

Herpes simplex is usually picked up by close contact with a carrier or someone who has an active herpes simplex lesion, usually a cold sore. The first infection in childhood is usually very severe. Often the child will present with severe painful crusting around the lips and mouth leading to an inability to eat or drink. Intravenous treatment may be required for this. Acyclovir is helpful, given systemically, in the amelioration of symptoms and in shortening the length of the attack. Topical cream must not be used in the mouth.

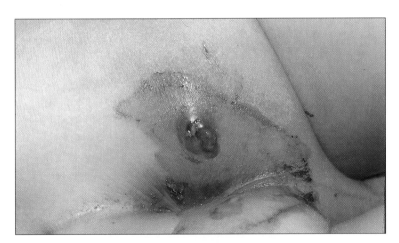

Figure 5.41
Discharging infection adjacent to the anus. This should be drained under general anesthetic and sigmoidoscopy performed to exclude anal fistulae. Inflammatory bowel disease also needs to be excluded.

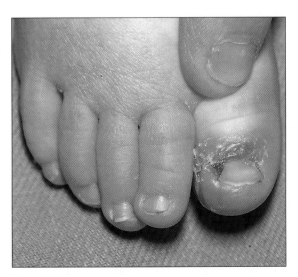

Figure 5.42
Ingrowing toe nail. There is little point in treating this with antibiotics. The nail is acting as a foreign body and as such needs to be removed before any treatment can begin.

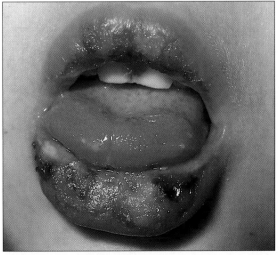

Figure 5.43
Herpes simplex infection of the lower lip. The child may need to be admitted if it is not possible for her to take fluids or nourishment orally.

Herpes simplex infection of the eye may result in a corneal ulcer developing (dendritic ulcer). If there is any doubt that a corneal lesion due to herpes simplex infection is present, the child should be referred immediately for expert ophthalmic opinion.

HERPETIC WHITLOW (Figure 5.44)
Herpetic lesions may be seen on the fingers of children who also have mouth lesions. It is rare for them to occur when there is no mouth lesion present either in the child or an adult carer. One must not confuse this with paronychia as incision and drainage will be of no benefit and may prolong the condition. Indeed, it may predispose to the development of superimposed bacterial infection.

FUNGAL INFECTIONS
THRUSH (CANDIDA) (Figure 5.45)
Candidal infections are common in young children. Typically, nappy rash presents with a red, angry perineum and buttocks with dotted satellite lesions over the body. In extreme cases the trunk and face can be completely covered with red angry lesions. In these situations the child should be admitted. Mild hydrocortisone cream may help take away the itching and irritation while nystatin ointment will help treat the underlying cause.

TINEAL INFECTIONS (Figure 5.47)
Athlete's foot and dhobie rash of the groin occur in teenage boys in whom hygiene may be suspect! More probably it is related to the increase in sweating which is associated with pubertal changes. Local application of antifungal cream is usually effective.

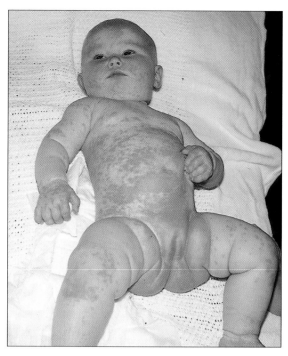

Figure 5.45
Diffuse seborrheic dermatitis. This is complicated by superimposed candidal infection.

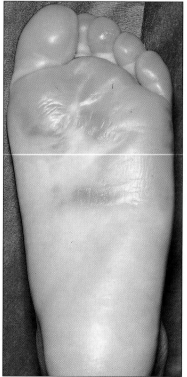

Figure 5.46
Athlete's foot in an adolescent male.

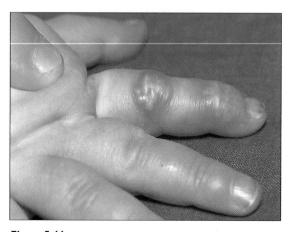

Figure 5.44
Herpetic whitlow. Picking at the lesions on her lip has led this child to a herpes simplex infection of the finger.

Index